Introduction

Welcome to **Healthy Cookbook For Athletes: 100 Recipes Balanced Meals for Strength, Stamina, and Speed!**

As an athlete, you understand that your body is your most valuable asset. Whether you're sprinting on the track, lifting weights in the gym, or competing on the field, the fuel you choose to power your body is just as important as your training regimen. This cookbook is designed to help you optimize your nutrition with 100 balanced, delicious recipes that support your goals for strength, stamina, and speed.

The meals and snacks within these pages are crafted to provide the essential nutrients you need for peak performance. You'll find a diverse array of recipes that cater to various dietary preferences and requirements, ensuring you can enjoy flavorful, nutritious meals that align with your individual needs. From protein-packed breakfasts to energy-boosting lunches, recovery-focused dinners, and snacks that keep you going, every recipe is designed to enhance your athletic performance and overall well-being.

We've focused on incorporating whole, nutrient-dense ingredients that provide a balanced mix of macronutrients—proteins for muscle repair and growth, carbohydrates for sustained energy, and healthy fats for endurance. Additionally, you'll find recipes rich in vitamins and minerals to support your immune system, reduce inflammation, and promote overall health.

In addition to the recipes, this cookbook offers practical tips on meal planning, preparation, and timing, helping you to seamlessly integrate these meals into your busy lifestyle. We've included guidance on what to eat before and after workouts, how to stay properly hydrated, and ways to make meal prep more efficient, so you can spend more time focusing on your training and less time worrying about what to eat.

Embark on this culinary journey to discover new ways to fuel your body and mind. With the right nutrition, you'll not only enhance your athletic performance but also develop sustainable eating habits that will benefit you throughout your life. Get ready to cook up a storm, fuel your passion, and achieve your goals with **Healthy Cookbook For Athletes: 100 Recipes Balanced Meals for Strength, Stamina, and Speed**.

Let's dive in and start fueling your body for success!

Warmest regards,

Daisy Robinson

Dear Valued Customer,

*Thank you for purchasing **Healthy Cookbook For Athletes: 100 Recipes Balanced Meals for Strength, Stamina, and Speed!***

We are delighted that you've chosen this book as a part of your journey towards peak performance and optimal health. Your commitment to fueling your body with nutritious, balanced meals is a crucial step towards achieving your athletic goals and maintaining a vibrant, energetic lifestyle.

Inside this cookbook, you'll find 100 recipes meticulously designed to enhance your strength, stamina, and speed. We hope these meals inspire you to explore new flavors and ingredients, making your nutrition journey as enjoyable as it is beneficial. Whether you're preparing meals for intense training days or looking for quick, healthy options on rest days, we believe you'll find recipes that become staples in your kitchen.

Your support means the world to us. We are here to cheer you on every step of the way, and we'd love to hear about your experiences with the recipes. If you have any feedback or questions, please don't hesitate to reach out.

*Thank you once again for choosing **Healthy Cookbook For Athletes.** Wishing you success, health, and happiness as you continue to fuel your passion and achieve your goals.*

Happy cooking!

Warmest regards,

Daisy Robinson
P.S. Don't forget to share your culinary creations and athletic achievements with us! We love seeing how our recipes contribute to your success.

1. Grilled chicken breast with quinoa and steamed vegetables

Ingredients:

For the chicken:

- 4 boneless, skinless chicken breasts
- 2 tablespoons olive oil
- 1 teaspoon paprika
- 1 teaspoon garlic powder
- Salt and pepper to taste

For the vegetables:

- 1 cup broccoli florets
- 1 cup cauliflower florets
- 1 cup sliced carrots
- 1 tablespoon olive oil
- Salt and pepper to taste

For the quinoa:

- 1 cup quinoa, rinsed
- 2 cups chicken broth or water
- 1 tablespoon lemon juice
- 2 tablespoons chopped fresh parsley

Instructions:

1. Preheat your grill or grill pan to medium-high heat.

2. Brush the chicken breasts with olive oil and season with paprika, garlic powder, salt, and pepper.

3. Grill the chicken breasts for about 6-8 minutes per side, or until cooked through. Set aside and let rest for 5 minutes before slicing.

4. In a saucepan, combine the quinoa and chicken broth (or water). Bring to a boil, then reduce heat to low, cover, and simmer for 15-20 minutes until the quinoa is tender and the liquid is absorbed. Fluff with a fork and stir in the lemon juice and parsley.

5. In a steamer basket, steam the broccoli, cauliflower, and carrots for 5-7 minutes until tender-crisp. Toss with olive oil, salt, and pepper.

6. To serve, divide the quinoa among plates, top with sliced grilled chicken, and arrange the steamed vegetables on the side.

This recipe provides a balanced meal with lean protein from the chicken, complex carbohydrates from the quinoa, and essential nutrients from the vegetables. It's a great option for athletes looking for a nutritious and satisfying meal to fuel their active lifestyle.

2. Baked salmon with sweet potato and asparagus

Ingredients:
For the salmon:
- 4 (6-ounce) salmon fillets
- 2 tablespoons olive oil
- Salt and pepper to taste
- 1 lemon, sliced into wedges

For the asparagus:
- 1 bunch asparagus, trimmed
- 2 tablespoons olive oil
- 2 cloves garlic, minced
- Salt and pepper to taste

For the sweet potato:
- 2 large sweet potatoes, peeled and cut into 1-inch cubes
- 2 tablespoons olive oil
- 1 teaspoon paprika
- Salt and pepper to taste

Instructions:
1. Preheat your oven to 400°F (200°C).

2. Prepare the salmon: Place the salmon fillets on a baking sheet lined with parchment paper or foil. Drizzle with olive oil and season with salt and pepper. Set aside.

3. Prepare the sweet potato: In a large bowl, toss the sweet potato cubes with olive oil, paprika, salt, and pepper until well coated. Spread the cubes in a single layer on a baking sheet.

4. Prepare the asparagus: In the same bowl, toss the asparagus with olive oil, minced garlic, salt, and pepper until well coated.

5. Place the salmon and sweet potato in the preheated oven. Bake for 15 minutes.

6. After 15 minutes, remove the baking sheet from the oven and add the asparagus to the same sheet as the sweet potato. Return to the oven and bake for another 10-15 minutes, or until the salmon is cooked through and the vegetables are tender.

7. Remove from the oven and serve hot, with lemon wedges on the side for squeezing over the salmon.

This recipe is packed with nutrients and provides a balanced combination of lean protein from the salmon, complex carbohydrates from the sweet potato, and fiber and vitamins from the asparagus. The healthy fats in the olive oil and salmon also contribute to the overall nutritional value of this meal, making it an excellent choice for athletes looking to fuel their bodies with wholesome, nourishing foods.

3. Turkey chili with beans and vegetables

Ingredients:
- 1 lb lean ground turkey
- 1 large onion, diced
- 3 cloves garlic, minced
- 2 bell peppers (any color), diced
- 2 carrots, diced
- 2 celery stalks, diced
- 1 (28 oz) can diced tomatoes
- 1 (15 oz) can kidney beans, drained and rinsed
- 1 (15 oz) can black beans, drained and rinsed
- 1 (6 oz) can tomato paste
- 2 cups vegetable or chicken broth
- 2 tablespoons chili powder
- 1 teaspoon ground cumin
- 1 teaspoon smoked paprika
- 1 teaspoon dried oregano
- Salt and pepper to taste
- Toppings (optional): shredded cheese, avocado, sour cream, chopped cilantro

Instructions:

1. In a large pot or Dutch oven, cook the ground turkey over medium-high heat until browned and crumbled, about 5-7 minutes. Drain any excess fat.

2. Add the onion, garlic, bell peppers, carrots, and celery to the pot. Cook for 5-7 minutes, stirring occasionally, until the vegetables are slightly softened.

3. Add the diced tomatoes (with their juices), kidney beans, black beans, tomato paste, broth, chili powder, cumin, smoked paprika, oregano, salt, and pepper. Stir to combine.

4. Bring the chili to a boil, then reduce the heat to low and let it simmer for 30-40 minutes, stirring occasionally, until the flavors have melded and the chili has thickened slightly.

5. Taste and adjust seasoning as needed, adding more salt, pepper, or other spices to your liking.

6. Serve the chili hot, garnished with desired toppings such as shredded cheese, avocado, sour cream, or chopped cilantro.

This turkey chili is packed with lean protein from the ground turkey, fiber from the beans and vegetables, and a variety of vitamins and minerals essential for an athlete's recovery and performance. The complex carbohydrates from the beans and vegetables provide sustained energy, while the spices add flavor and potential anti-inflammatory benefits. Adjust the spiciness level to your preference, and feel free to add or substitute other vegetables you enjoy. This hearty and nutritious chili is sure to satisfy and fuel your active lifestyle.

4. Brown rice stir-fry with tofu and mixed vegetables

Ingredients:
- 3 cloves garlic, minced
- 1 tablespoon freshly grated ginger
- 3 tablespoons low-sodium soy sauce
- 2 tablespoons rice vinegar
- 1 tablespoon honey or maple syrup
- 1 teaspoon sesame seeds (optional garnish)
- Sliced green onions (optional garnish)
- 1 cup brown rice, cooked according to package instructions
- 1 (14 oz) block extra-firm tofu, drained and cut into 1-inch cubes
- 2 tablespoons sesame oil or vegetable oil
- 1 cup broccoli florets
- 1 cup sliced carrots
- 1 cup sliced bell pepper (any color)
- 1 cup snow peas or sugar snap peas

Instructions:

1. Cook the brown rice according to package instructions. Set aside.

2. In a large skillet or wok, heat 1 tablespoon of sesame oil or vegetable oil over medium-high heat. Add the tofu cubes and stir-fry for 5-7 minutes until lightly browned. Remove the tofu from the skillet and set aside.

3. In the same skillet, add the remaining 1 tablespoon of oil. Add the broccoli, carrots, bell pepper, and snow peas or sugar snap peas. Stir-fry for 5-7 minutes until the vegetables are tender-crisp.

4. Add the minced garlic and grated ginger to the skillet and cook for 1 minute, stirring constantly, until fragrant.

5. In a small bowl, whisk together the soy sauce, rice vinegar, and honey or maple syrup.

6. Return the cooked tofu to the skillet with the vegetables. Add the cooked brown rice and the soy sauce mixture. Toss everything together gently until well combined and heated through.

7. Remove from heat and garnish with sesame seeds and sliced green onions, if desired.

This stir-fry is packed with plant-based protein from the tofu, complex carbohydrates from the brown rice, and an abundance of vitamins, minerals, and fiber from the mixed vegetables. The combination of flavors from the soy sauce, rice vinegar, and honey or maple syrup adds a delicious umami taste. This dish is a great option for athletes looking for a balanced and satisfying meal that provides sustained energy and essential nutrients for recovery and performance.

5. Whole wheat pasta with lean ground turkey and marinara sauce

1. Whole wheat pasta:

- Provides complex carbohydrates, which are an essential source of energy for athletes.

- Whole grains are rich in fiber, which aids digestion and helps maintain a healthy gut.

- Whole grains also offer various vitamins and minerals, such as B vitamins, iron, and magnesium.

2. Lean ground turkey:

- A great source of lean protein, which is crucial for muscle repair and recovery after intense workouts.

- Turkey is lower in saturated fat compared to other red meats, making it a healthier choice.

- Protein helps athletes feel fuller for longer, preventing overeating.

3. Marinara sauce:

- Tomato-based sauces are rich in various antioxidants, such as lycopene, which can help reduce inflammation.

- The sauce can provide additional nutrients, such as vitamin C, vitamin K, and potassium, depending on the ingredients used.

To make this meal even more nutritious for athletes, consider adding some vegetables, such as sautéed spinach, bell peppers, or zucchini, to increase the fiber, vitamin, and mineral content. You could also top the dish with a sprinkle of Parmesan cheese for an additional protein boost.

Overall, this meal provides a good balance of complex carbohydrates, lean protein, and essential nutrients, making it a suitable choice for athletes seeking to fuel their bodies and support recovery after intense physical activities.

6. Grilled shrimp skewers with roasted vegetables

Ingredients:
For the Shrimp Skewers:
- 1 lb large shrimp, peeled and deveined
- 2 tbsp olive oil
- 2 cloves garlic, minced
- 1 tsp paprika
- 1/2 tsp dried oregano
- Juice of 1 lemon
- Salt and pepper to taste

For the Roasted Vegetables:
- 1 zucchini, sliced into rounds
- 1 red bell pepper, cut into chunks
- 1 red onion, cut into wedges
- 1 cup cherry tomatoes
- 2 tbsp olive oil
- 2 cloves garlic, minced
- Salt and pepper to taste

Instructions:
1. Preheat your grill to medium-high heat and preheat your oven to 400°F (200°C).

2. In a bowl, toss the shrimp with olive oil, garlic, paprika, oregano, lemon juice, salt, and pepper. Thread the shrimp onto skewers.

3. On a large baking sheet, toss the zucchini, bell pepper, onion, and cherry tomatoes with olive oil, garlic, salt, and pepper.

4. Roast the vegetables in the preheated oven for 20-25 minutes, tossing halfway through, until tender and slightly charred.

5. Grill the shrimp skewers for 2-3 minutes per side, or until the shrimp are opaque and cooked through.

6. Serve the grilled shrimp skewers with the roasted vegetables on the side.

This meal provides a great balance of lean protein from the shrimp, complex carbohydrates from the vegetables, and essential vitamins, minerals, and antioxidants. The grilling and roasting methods also add a delicious smoky flavor while keeping the meal relatively low in fat. Enjoy this flavorful and nutritious dish to fuel your athletic endeavors!

7. Greek yogurt parfait with granola and mixed berries

Ingredients:
- **1** cup plain Greek yogurt
- (high-protein variety, if possible)
- 1/2 cup mixed berries
- (such as strawberries, blueberries, raspberries)
- 1/4 cup homemade granola (see recipe below)
- 1 tbsp chia seeds or flaxseeds (optional)
- 1 tsp honey or maple syrup (optional)

Homemade Granola:
- 2 cups old-fashioned oats
- 1/4 cup sliced almonds or chopped nuts of your choice
- 2 tbsp chia seeds or flaxseeds
- 2 tbsp honey or maple syrup
- 1 tbsp coconut oil, melted
- 1 tsp vanilla extract
- 1/4 tsp ground cinnamon
- Pinch of salt

Instructions:

1. Preheat your oven to 325°F (165°C).

2. To make the granola, mix the oats, nuts, chia/flaxseeds, honey/maple syrup, coconut oil, vanilla, cinnamon, and salt in a bowl until well combined.

3. Spread the granola mixture onto a baking sheet lined with parchment paper.

4. Bake for 20-25 minutes, stirring occasionally, until the granola is golden brown and fragrant.

5. Remove the granola from the oven and let it cool completely. To assemble the parfait, layer half of the Greek yogurt into a glass or jar.

6. Top with half of the mixed berries and half of the granola. Repeat the layers with the remaining yogurt, berries, and granola.

7. Optionally, sprinkle with chia/flaxseeds and drizzle with a teaspoon of honey or maple syrup for added sweetness.

This parfait provides a balanced combination of protein from the Greek yogurt, complex carbohydrates and fiber from the oats and berries, and healthy fats from the nuts and seeds. The chia/flaxseeds add an extra boost of omega-3 fatty acids, which can help reduce inflammation and support recovery.

The homemade granola is a healthier option than store-bought varieties, as it's free from added sugars and preservatives. You can also customize the granola recipe by adding your favorite nuts, seeds, or dried fruits.

This parfait makes for a delicious and nutritious breakfast, snack, or post-workout meal for athletes, providing sustained energy and supporting muscle recovery and overall health.

8. Quinoa salad with black beans, corn, and avocado

Ingredients:
- 1 cup uncooked quinoa
- 1 (15 oz) can black beans, rinsed and drained
- 1 cup frozen corn kernels, thawed
- 1 avocado, diced
- 1/2 red onion, diced
- 1 jalapeño, seeded and minced (optional, for a kick of heat)
- 1/4 cup fresh cilantro, chopped
- Juice of 1 lime
- 2 tbsp olive oil
- 1 tsp ground cumin
- Salt and pepper to taste

Instructions:
1. Cook the quinoa according to package instructions. Fluff with a fork and set aside to cool.

2. In a large bowl, combine the cooled quinoa, black beans, corn, avocado, red onion, jalapeño (if using), and cilantro.

3. In a small bowl, whisk together the lime juice, olive oil, cumin, salt, and pepper. Pour the dressing over the quinoa salad and gently toss to combine.

4. Taste and adjust seasoning if needed. Cover and refrigerate for at least 30 minutes before serving to allow the flavors to meld.

This quinoa salad is packed with nutrients that are beneficial for athletes:

- Quinoa is a complete protein source, providing all the essential amino acids needed for muscle repair and growth.
- Black beans are high in protein and fiber, which helps promote feelings of fullness and sustained energy.
- Corn provides complex carbohydrates for energy, as well as antioxidants like lutein and zeaxanthin.
- Avocado offers healthy monounsaturated fats, potassium, and fiber.
- The combination of veggies and herbs provides a variety of vitamins, minerals, and antioxidants to support overall health and recovery.

This salad can be enjoyed as a main dish or a side, and it's perfect for meal prepping or packing for a post-workout meal. The flavors and textures blend beautifully, making it a delicious and satisfying option for athletes seeking a nutritious and protein-packed meal.

9. Baked chicken thighs with roasted Brussels sprouts and butternut squash

Ingredients:
- 8 bone-in, skin-on chicken thighs
- 2 tbsp olive oil, divided
- 1 tsp salt
- 1/2 tsp black pepper
- 1 tsp paprika
- 1 tsp dried thyme
- 1 lb Brussels sprouts, trimmed and halved
- 2 cups cubed butternut squash (about 1/2 medium squash)
- 2 cloves garlic, minced
- 2 tbsp balsamic vinegar

Instructions:

1. Preheat your oven to 400°F (200°C).

2. Pat the chicken thighs dry with paper towels and place them in a large baking dish or rimmed baking sheet. Drizzle with 1 tablespoon of olive oil and season with salt, black pepper, paprika, and dried thyme. Rub the seasoning all over the chicken.

3. On a separate baking sheet, toss the Brussels sprouts and cubed butternut squash with the remaining 1 tablespoon of olive oil, minced garlic, salt, and pepper.

4. Roast the chicken thighs and the vegetables in the preheated oven. The chicken will take about 35-40 minutes to cook through, while the vegetables will need 25-30 minutes, tossing them halfway through.

5. Once the vegetables are tender and caramelized, remove them from the oven and drizzle with balsamic vinegar. Toss to coat evenly.

6. Serve the baked chicken thighs alongside the roasted Brussels sprouts and butternut squash.

This meal is an excellent choice for athletes because:

- Chicken thighs are a great source of lean protein, essential for muscle repair and recovery.
- Brussels sprouts and butternut squash are nutrient-dense vegetables, providing complex carbohydrates, fiber, vitamins, and minerals.
- Olive oil and balsamic vinegar offer healthy fats and antioxidants.
- The combination of protein, complex carbs, and veggies makes for a well-balanced, satisfying meal.

The baking method ensures that the chicken stays moist and juicy, while the vegetables develop a delicious caramelized flavor. This meal is easy to prepare and can be enjoyed after a workout or as part of a meal prep plan for athletes. Adjust the portion sizes according to your individual caloric and nutrient needs.

10. Veggie omelette with spinach, tomatoes, and mushrooms

Ingredients:
- 3 large eggs
- 2 tbsp milk (or plant-based milk alternative)
- 1/4 tsp salt
- 1 tsp olive oil
- 1/4 tsp black pepper
- 1 cup fresh spinach, roughly chopped
- 1/2 cup sliced mushrooms
- 1/2 cup diced tomatoes
- 2 tbsp crumbled feta cheese (optional)

Instructions:

1. Crack the eggs into a small bowl, add the milk, salt, and pepper. Whisk well until the mixture is smooth and slightly frothy. Heat the olive oil in a non-stick skillet over medium heat.

2. Add the chopped spinach, sliced mushrooms, and diced tomatoes to the skillet. Sauté for 2-3 minutes, or until the vegetables are slightly softened.

3. Pour the egg mixture over the vegetables, tilting the pan to evenly distribute the eggs.

4. As the eggs start to set around the edges, use a spatula to gently lift the edges and tilt the pan to allow the uncooked egg to flow underneath.

5. When the omelette is almost set but still a bit runny on top, sprinkle the feta cheese (if using) over one half of the omelette. Fold the other half of the omelette over the filling and slide it onto a plate.

This veggie omelette is an excellent choice for athletes for several reasons:

- Eggs are a high-quality protein source, essential for muscle repair and recovery after intense workouts.
- Spinach is rich in iron, which is important for oxygen transport and energy production.
- Tomatoes are a good source of vitamin C, an antioxidant that can help reduce exercise-induced oxidative stress.
- Mushrooms are a good source of B vitamins, which are essential for energy metabolism.
- The addition of feta cheese provides a source of calcium, which is important for bone health and muscle function.

This omelette is also low in calories and high in nutrients, making it a great option for athletes trying to maintain a healthy weight while meeting their nutritional needs.

You can serve this veggie omelette with whole-grain toast or a side of fresh fruit for additional carbohydrates and fiber. It's a versatile meal that can be enjoyed for breakfast, lunch, or a post-workout snack.

11. Lentil soup with whole grain bread

Ingredients:
For the Lentil Soup:
- 1 cup dried green or brown lentils, rinsed
- 1 tbsp olive oil
- 1 onion, diced
- 2 carrots, diced
- 2 cloves garlic, minced
- 1 tsp ground cumin
- 1/2 tsp dried thyme
- 2 celery stalks, diced
- 4 cups vegetable or chicken broth
- 2 cups water
- Salt and pepper to taste
- Lemon wedges for serving

For the Whole Grain Bread:
4-6 slices of your favorite whole grain bread

Instructions:
1. In a large pot or Dutch oven, heat the olive oil over medium heat. Add the diced onion, carrots, and celery. Cook for 5-7 minutes until the vegetables are softened.

2. Add the minced garlic, cumin, and thyme. Cook for 1 minute until fragrant. Add the rinsed lentils, broth, and water to the pot. Season with salt and pepper to taste.

3. Bring the soup to a boil, then reduce the heat to low. Simmer for 20-25 minutes, or until the lentils are tender.

4. Adjust seasoning if needed and add a squeeze of lemon juice to brighten the flavors. Serve the lentil soup hot, with slices of whole grain bread on the side.

This lentil soup and whole grain bread combination is an excellent choice for athletes for several reasons:
- Lentils are a great source of plant-based protein, fiber, and complex carbohydrates, providing sustained energy and aiding in muscle recovery.
- The vegetables in the soup offer a variety of vitamins, minerals, and antioxidants essential for overall health and performance.
- Whole grain bread provides additional complex carbohydrates, fiber, and various nutrients like B vitamins and minerals.
- The combination of lentils, vegetables, and whole grains creates a well-balanced meal with a good mix of protein, carbs, and fiber.
- The soup is easy to digest and can be a comforting meal after intense workouts or training sessions.

You can adjust the portion sizes based on your individual caloric and nutrient needs. This meal is also highly customizable; you can add additional vegetables, herbs, or spices to suit your taste preferences. The lentil soup can be made in advance and reheated, making it a convenient option for meal prepping.

12. Grilled steak with roasted cauliflower and broccoli

Ingredients:
For the Steak:
- 1 lb (454g) flank steak or
your preferred cut of steak
- 2 tbsp olive oil
- 1 tsp salt
- 1/2 tsp black pepper
- 1 tsp dried thyme (optional)

For the Roasted Vegetables:
- 1 small head of cauliflower, cut into florets
- 1 large head of broccoli, cut into florets
- 2 tbsp olive oil
- 2 cloves garlic, minced
- 1 tsp paprika
- Salt and pepper to taste

Instructions:

1. Preheat your grill to high heat (or preheat your oven to 400°F/200°C if you prefer to broil the steak).

2. Pat the steak dry with paper towels and rub it with olive oil, salt, pepper, and dried thyme (if using). In a large bowl, toss the cauliflower and broccoli florets with olive oil, minced garlic, paprika, salt, and pepper until well coated.

3. Spread the vegetables in a single layer on a large baking sheet lined with foil or parchment paper.

4. Roast the vegetables in the preheated oven for 20-25 minutes, tossing them halfway through, until tender and lightly charred.

5. While the vegetables are roasting, grill the steak for 3-5 minutes per side (for medium-rare), or until it reaches your desired doneness. Let the steak rest for 5 minutes before slicing against the grain. Serve the grilled steak alongside the roasted cauliflower and broccoli.

This meal is an excellent choice for athletes because:
- Steak is a high-quality source of protein, essential for muscle repair and recovery after intense workouts.
- Cauliflower and broccoli are nutrient-dense vegetables that provide complex carbohydrates, fiber, vitamins, and minerals.
- Olive oil is a healthy fat source that aids in nutrient absorption and provides energy.
- The combination of lean protein, complex carbs, and vegetables creates a well-balanced meal that can support athletic performance and recovery.

This meal is also versatile; you can switch up the vegetable options or try different seasoning blends to keep things interesting. Enjoy this flavorful and nutritious meal as a post-workout refuel or as part of your overall balanced diet for athletic performance.

13. Turkey and vegetable kebabs with couscous

Ingredients:
For the kebabs:
- 1 lb (450g) turkey breast, cut into chunks
- 1 red bell pepper, cut into chunks
- 1 yellow bell pepper, cut into chunks
- 1 red onion, cut into chunks
- 1 zucchini, sliced into rounds
- 1 tablespoon olive oil
- 2 cloves garlic, minced
- 1 teaspoon dried oregano
- Salt and pepper to taste
- Wooden skewers, soaked in water for 30 minutes

For the couscous:
- 1 cup couscous
- 1 1/4 cups chicken or vegetable broth
- 1 tablespoon olive oil
- Salt and pepper to taste
- 2 tablespoons chopped fresh parsley

Instructions:

1. Preheat your grill to medium-high heat.

2. In a bowl, combine the olive oil, minced garlic, dried oregano, salt, and pepper. Add the turkey chunks and vegetables to the bowl and toss until they are evenly coated with the marinade.

3. Thread the marinated turkey and vegetables onto the soaked wooden skewers, alternating between each ingredient.

4. Place the kebabs on the preheated grill and cook for about 8-10 minutes, turning occasionally, until the turkey is cooked through and the vegetables are tender and slightly charred.

5. While the kebabs are cooking, prepare the couscous. In a saucepan, bring the chicken or vegetable broth to a boil. Stir in the couscous, cover the saucepan, and remove it from the heat. Let it sit for about 5 minutes, until the couscous has absorbed all the liquid. Fluff the couscous with a fork and stir in the olive oil, salt, pepper, and chopped parsley.

6. Serve the turkey and vegetable kebabs hot off the grill with a side of the fluffy couscous.

Enjoy your nutritious and protein-packed meal, perfect for athletes looking for a delicious and satisfying option!

14. Stuffed bell peppers with ground turkey and brown rice

Ingredients:
- 4 large bell peppers (any color), tops cut off and seeds removed
- 1 lb (450g) ground turkey
- 1 cup cooked brown rice
- 1 small onion, finely chopped
- 2 cloves garlic, minced
- 1 can (14.5 oz) diced tomatoes, drained
- 1 teaspoon dried oregano
- 1 teaspoon dried basil
- 1 teaspoon paprika
- 1/2 teaspoon salt
- 1/2 teaspoon black pepper
- 1/2 cup shredded mozzarella or cheddar cheese (optional)
- 1 tablespoon olive oil
- Fresh parsley or cilantro, chopped (for garnish)

Instructions:

1. Preheat your oven to 375°F (190°C).

2. In a large skillet, heat the olive oil over medium heat. Add the chopped onion and garlic, and sauté until they are softened and fragrant, about 3-4 minutes.

3. Add the ground turkey to the skillet and cook until it is browned and cooked through, breaking it up with a spoon as it cooks.

4. Stir in the diced tomatoes, cooked brown rice, dried oregano, dried basil, paprika, salt, and pepper. Cook for another 5 minutes, until everything is well combined and heated through.

5. Remove the skillet from the heat and let the filling cool slightly.

6. Stuff each bell pepper with the turkey and rice mixture, pressing down gently to pack the filling in.

7. Place the stuffed peppers upright in a baking dish. If you like, sprinkle the tops with shredded cheese.

8. Cover the baking dish with aluminum foil and bake in the preheated oven for 30 minutes. Remove the foil and bake for an additional 10-15 minutes, until the peppers are tender and the cheese (if used) is melted and bubbly.

9. Remove the stuffed peppers from the oven and let them cool slightly before serving. Garnish with chopped fresh parsley or cilantro.

Enjoy your healthy and delicious stuffed bell peppers, perfect for athletes needing a balanced and nutritious meal!

15. Baked cod with quinoa pilaf and steamed green beans

Ingredients:
For the baked cod:
- 4 cod fillets (about 6 oz each)
- 2 tablespoons olive oil
- 2 cloves garlic, minced
- 1 teaspoon paprika
- 1 teaspoon dried thyme
- Salt and pepper to taste
- Lemon wedges, for serving

For the quinoa pilaf:
- 1 cup quinoa, rinsed
- 2 cups vegetable or chicken broth
- 1 tablespoon olive oil
- 1 small onion, finely chopped
- 2 cloves garlic, minced
- 1 carrot, diced
- 1/2 cup frozen peas
- 1/4 cup chopped fresh parsley
- Salt and pepper to taste

Instructions:

1. Preheat your oven to 375°F (190°C).

For the steamed green beans:
- 1 lb (450g) green beans, trimmed
- Salt to taste

2. In a small bowl, mix together the olive oil, minced garlic, paprika, dried thyme, salt, and pepper.

3. Place the cod fillets on a baking sheet lined with parchment paper. Brush each fillet with the olive oil mixture, making sure to coat both sides.

4. Bake the cod in the preheated oven for 12-15 minutes, or until the fish flakes easily with a fork.

5. While the cod is baking, prepare the quinoa pilaf. In a medium saucepan, heat the olive oil over medium heat. Add the chopped onion and garlic, and sauté until they are softened and fragrant, about 3-4 minutes.

6. Add the quinoa to the saucepan and toast it for a couple of minutes, stirring frequently.

7. Pour in the vegetable or chicken broth and bring the mixture to a boil. Reduce the heat to low, cover the saucepan, and let the quinoa simmer for about 15 minutes, or until all the liquid is absorbed and the quinoa is cooked through.

8. In the meantime, steam the green beans until they are tender yet still crisp, about 5-7 minutes. Season with salt to taste.

9. Once the quinoa is cooked, fluff it with a fork and stir in the diced carrot, frozen peas, chopped parsley, salt, and pepper. Cover the saucepan and let it sit for a few minutes to allow the vegetables to warm through.

10. Serve the baked cod with a generous scoop of quinoa pilaf and steamed green beans on the side. Garnish with lemon wedges for squeezing over the fish.

16. Chickpea salad with cucumber, tomatoes, and feta cheese

Ingredients:
- 2 cans (15 oz each) chickpeas, drained and rinsed
- 1 cucumber, diced
- 1 pint cherry tomatoes, halved
- 1/2 cup crumbled feta cheese
- 1/4 cup chopped fresh parsley
- 1/4 cup chopped fresh mint
- 1/4 cup extra virgin olive oil
- 2 tablespoons lemon juice
- 2 cloves garlic, minced
- Salt and pepper to taste

Instructions:

1. In a large mixing bowl, combine the chickpeas, diced cucumber, halved cherry tomatoes, crumbled feta cheese, chopped fresh parsley, and chopped fresh mint.

2. In a small bowl, whisk together the extra virgin olive oil, lemon juice, minced garlic, salt, and pepper to make the dressing.

3. Pour the dressing over the chickpea salad and toss gently until everything is well coated.

4. Taste and adjust the seasoning if needed, adding more salt, pepper, or lemon juice to your preference.

5. Cover the bowl with plastic wrap or transfer the salad to an airtight container and refrigerate for at least 30 minutes to allow the flavors to meld together.

6. Serve the chickpea salad chilled as a refreshing and nutritious meal or side dish.

This chickpea salad is packed with protein, fiber, and vitamins, making it an excellent choice for athletes looking for a light yet satisfying option to fuel their bodies. Enjoy!

17. Grilled pork tenderloin with roasted sweet potatoes and zucchini

Ingredients:

For the pork tenderloin:
- 2 pork tenderloins (about 1 lb each)
- 2 tablespoons olive oil
- 2 cloves garlic, minced
- 1 teaspoon dried thyme
- 1 teaspoon paprika
- Salt and pepper to taste

For the roasted sweet potatoes and zucchini:
- 2 large sweet potatoes, peeled and cubed
- 2 medium zucchini, sliced into rounds
- 2 tablespoons olive oil
- 1 teaspoon garlic powder
- 1 teaspoon dried rosemary
- Salt and pepper to taste

Instructions:

1. Preheat your grill to medium-high heat.

2. In a small bowl, mix together the olive oil, minced garlic, dried thyme, paprika, salt, and pepper to create a marinade for the pork tenderloins.

3. Rub the marinade all over the pork tenderloins, coating them evenly. Let them marinate for at least 30 minutes to allow the flavors to penetrate the meat.

4. While the pork is marinating, preheat your oven to 400°F (200°C) and prepare a baking sheet lined with parchment paper.

5. In a large mixing bowl, toss the cubed sweet potatoes and sliced zucchini with olive oil, garlic powder, dried rosemary, salt, and pepper until they are well coated.

6. Spread the sweet potatoes and zucchini in a single layer on the prepared baking sheet.

7. Roast the sweet potatoes and zucchini in the preheated oven for 20-25 minutes, or until they are tender and slightly caramelized, stirring halfway through cooking.

8. While the vegetables are roasting, grill the marinated pork tenderloins on the preheated grill for about 15-20 minutes, turning occasionally, until they are cooked through and have reached an internal temperature of 145°F (63°C).

9. Remove the pork tenderloins from the grill and let them rest for a few minutes before slicing them into thick slices. Serve the grilled pork tenderloin slices with the roasted sweet potatoes and zucchini on the side.

This hearty and nutritious meal provides a balanced combination of protein, carbohydrates, and vegetables, making it ideal for athletes needing to refuel and replenish after a workout. Enjoy!

18. Spinach and feta turkey burgers with whole wheat buns

Ingredients:
For the turkey burgers:
- 1 lb (450g) lean ground turkey
- 1 cup fresh spinach, chopped
- 1/2 cup crumbled feta cheese
- 2 cloves garlic, minced
- 1/4 cup finely chopped red onion
- 1 teaspoon dried oregano
- 1 teaspoon dried basil
- Salt and pepper to taste
- Olive oil for cooking

For serving:
- Whole wheat burger buns
- Lettuce leaves
- Sliced tomatoes
- Sliced red onion
- Avocado slices (optional)

Instructions:

1. In a large mixing bowl, combine the ground turkey, chopped spinach, crumbled feta cheese, minced garlic, chopped red onion, dried oregano, dried basil, salt, and pepper. Mix until all the ingredients are well incorporated.

2. Divide the turkey mixture into 4 equal portions and shape each portion into a burger patty.

3. Preheat a grill or grill pan over medium-high heat. Brush the grill grates or pan with a little olive oil to prevent sticking.

4. Place the turkey burgers on the preheated grill or grill pan and cook for about 5-6 minutes per side, or until they are cooked through and no longer pink in the center.

5. While the burgers are cooking, toast the whole wheat burger buns on the grill for a minute or two until they are lightly golden brown.

6. Assemble the burgers by placing a turkey burger patty on each toasted bun. Top with lettuce leaves, sliced tomatoes, sliced red onion, and avocado slices if desired.

7. Serve the spinach and feta turkey burgers immediately, accompanied by your favorite side dishes or a fresh salad.

These turkey burgers are packed with lean protein and wholesome ingredients, making them a nutritious and satisfying option for athletes looking to refuel after a workout. Enjoy!

19. Mixed bean salad with bell peppers, onions, and a lemon vinaigrette

Ingredients:
For the salad:
- 1 can (15 oz) black beans, drained and rinsed
- 1 can (15 oz) kidney beans, drained and rinsed
- 1 can (15 oz) chickpeas (garbanzo beans), drained and rinsed
- 1 red bell pepper, diced
- 1 yellow bell pepper, diced
- 1/2 red onion, finely chopped
- 1/4 cup chopped fresh parsley
- Salt and pepper to taste

For the lemon vinaigrette:
- 1/4 cup extra virgin olive oil
- Juice of 1 lemon
- 1 teaspoon Dijon mustard
- 1 clove garlic, minced
- 1 teaspoon honey or maple syrup (optional)
- Salt and pepper to taste

Instructions:

1. In a large mixing bowl, combine the drained and rinsed black beans, kidney beans, and chickpeas.

2. Add the diced red bell pepper, diced yellow bell pepper, finely chopped red onion, and chopped fresh parsley to the bowl with the beans.

3. Season the salad with salt and pepper to taste and toss gently to combine all the ingredients.

4. In a small bowl or measuring cup, whisk together the extra virgin olive oil, lemon juice, Dijon mustard, minced garlic, honey or maple syrup (if using), salt, and pepper to make the lemon vinaigrette.

5. Pour the lemon vinaigrette over the mixed bean salad and toss until everything is well coated in the dressing.

6. Taste and adjust the seasoning if needed, adding more salt, pepper, or lemon juice to your preference.

7. Cover the bowl with plastic wrap or transfer the salad to an airtight container and refrigerate for at least 30 minutes to allow the flavors to meld together.

8. Serve the mixed bean salad chilled as a nutritious and protein-rich meal or side dish.

This mixed bean salad is loaded with fiber, vitamins, and minerals, making it an excellent choice for athletes needing a healthy and satisfying option to support their training. Enjoy!

20. Baked tofu with stir-fried vegetables and brown rice

Ingredients:
For the baked tofu:
- 1 block (14 oz) extra firm tofu, pressed and drained
- 2 tablespoons soy sauce
- 1 tablespoon sesame oil
- 1 tablespoon maple syrup or honey
- 1 teaspoon garlic powder
- 1 teaspoon ground ginger
- 1 tablespoon cornstarch
- Salt and pepper to taste

For the stir-fried vegetables:
- 2 tablespoons vegetable oil
- 2 cups mixed vegetables (such as bell peppers, broccoli, carrots, snap peas)
- 2 cloves garlic, minced
- 1 tablespoon grated fresh ginger
- 2 tablespoons soy sauce
- 1 tablespoon hoisin sauce
- 1 teaspoon sesame oil
- Salt and pepper to taste

For serving: Cooked brown rice

Instructions:

1. Preheat your oven to 400°F (200°C). Line a baking sheet with parchment paper or lightly grease it. Cut the pressed tofu into cubes or strips, depending on your preference.

2. In a bowl, whisk together the soy sauce, sesame oil, maple syrup or honey, garlic powder, ground ginger, cornstarch (if using), salt, and pepper. Add the tofu cubes to the bowl and gently toss until they are evenly coated with the marinade.

3. Arrange the tofu cubes in a single layer on the prepared baking sheet. Bake in the preheated oven for 25-30 minutes, flipping halfway through, until the tofu is golden and crispy on the outside.

4. While the tofu is baking, prepare the stir-fried vegetables. Heat the vegetable oil in a large skillet or wok over medium-high heat.

5. Add the mixed vegetables to the skillet and stir-fry for 4-5 minutes, or until they are tender-crisp. Stir in the minced garlic and grated ginger, and cook for another minute until fragrant.

6. Add the soy sauce, hoisin sauce, sesame oil, salt, and pepper to the skillet, and toss everything together until the vegetables are evenly coated in the sauce. Serve the baked tofu and stir-fried vegetables over cooked brown rice.

This nutritious and flavorful dish provides a balanced combination of protein, carbohydrates, and vegetables, making it an ideal choice for athletes seeking a wholesome and satisfying meal. Enjoy!

21. Spaghetti squash with turkey meatballs and marinara sauce

Ingredients:
- 1 large spaghetti squash
- Olive oil, salt, and pepper
- 1 lb (450g) lean ground turkey
- 1/4 cup breadcrumbs
- 1/4 cup grated Parmesan cheese
- 1 egg
- 2 cloves garlic, minced
- 1 tsp each dried oregano and basil

For the marinara sauce:
1. 2 tbsp olive oil
2. 1 onion, minced
3. 2 cloves garlic, minced
4. 1 can (28 oz) crushed tomatoes
5. 1 tsp each dried oregano and basil
6. Salt and pepper to taste

Instructions:

1. Preheat oven to 400°F (200°C). Cut squash in half, scoop seeds, drizzle with olive oil, salt, and pepper. Roast cut side down for 40-50 mins.

2. Mix turkey, breadcrumbs, Parmesan, egg, garlic, oregano, basil. Form into meatballs.

3. Cook meatballs in olive oil until browned and cooked through.

4. Sauté onion and garlic in olive oil. Add crushed tomatoes, oregano, basil, salt, and pepper. Simmer.

5. Scrape squash into strands. Serve topped with meatballs and marinara sauce.

This dish is a delicious and nutritious alternative to traditional pasta, providing plenty of fiber, lean protein, and vitamins for athletes looking to fuel their bodies with wholesome ingredients. Enjoy!

22. Grilled chicken Caesar salad with whole grain croutons

Ingredients:
For the Caesar dressing:
- 1/3 cup mayonnaise
- 2 tablespoons grated Parmesan cheese
- 1 tablespoon lemon juice
- 1 clove garlic, minced
- 1 teaspoon Dijon mustard
- Salt and pepper to taste
- Water (optional, for thinning)

For the grilled chicken:
- 2 boneless, skinless chicken breasts
- 2 tablespoons olive oil
- 2 cloves garlic, minced
- 1 teaspoon dried oregano
- Salt and pepper to taste

For the salad:
- 1 head romaine lettuce, washed and chopped
- 1/4 cup grated Parmesan cheese
- Whole grain croutons (store-bought or homemade)

Instructions:
1. Preheat your grill to medium-high heat.

2. In a small bowl, mix together the olive oil, minced garlic, dried oregano, salt, and pepper to create a marinade for the chicken breasts.

3. Brush the chicken breasts with the marinade, coating them evenly.

4. Grill the chicken breasts for about 6-8 minutes per side, or until they are cooked through and no longer pink in the center. Remove from the grill and let them rest for a few minutes before slicing.

5. While the chicken is grilling, prepare the Caesar dressing. In a bowl, whisk together the mayonnaise, grated Parmesan cheese, lemon juice, minced garlic, Dijon mustard, salt, and pepper. If the dressing is too thick, you can thin it out with a little water.

6. In a large salad bowl, toss the chopped romaine lettuce with the grated Parmesan cheese and whole grain croutons.

7. Add the sliced grilled chicken on top of the salad. Drizzle the Caesar dressing over the salad or serve it on the side.

9. Toss the salad gently to coat everything in the dressing. Serve the grilled chicken Caesar salad immediately, garnished with extra Parmesan cheese and cracked black pepper if desired.

Enjoy this protein-packed and nutritious salad, perfect for athletes needing a satisfying and flavorful meal!

23. Teriyaki salmon with brown rice and steamed broccoli

Ingredients:
- 4 (6 oz) salmon fillets
- 1/4 cup low-sodium teriyaki sauce
- 1 cup uncooked brown rice
- 2 cups broccoli florets
- 1 tbsp olive oil
- Salt and pepper to taste

Instructions:
1. Preheat your oven to 400°F.

2. Place the salmon fillets in a baking dish and brush the top of each fillet with the teriyaki sauce.

3. Bake the salmon for 12-15 minutes, or until it flakes easily with a fork.

4. While the salmon is baking, cook the brown rice according to package instructions.

5. In a steamer basket, steam the broccoli florets for 5-7 minutes, until tender-crisp.

6. Serve the baked teriyaki salmon over the cooked brown rice, accompanied by the steamed broccoli.

7. Drizzle any remaining teriyaki sauce from the baking dish over the salmon and rice, if desired. Season the dish with salt and pepper to taste.

This recipe is an excellent choice for athletes for several reasons:

- Salmon is a high-quality protein source that is rich in omega-3 fatty acids, which can help reduce inflammation and support muscle recovery.
- Brown rice provides complex carbohydrates to fuel your workouts.
- Broccoli is a nutrient-dense vegetable that offers fiber, vitamins, and minerals.
- The teriyaki sauce adds flavor without excessive sodium or sugar.

This meal is well-balanced, providing a combination of lean protein, complex carbs, and essential nutrients to support an active lifestyle. The simplicity of the recipe also makes it easy to prepare, making it a great option for busy athletes.

Feel free to adjust the portion sizes or add additional vegetables to suit your individual needs. Enjoy this teriyaki salmon with brown rice and steamed broccoli as part of a healthy, athlete-friendly diet.

24. Turkey and vegetable stir-fry with quinoa

Ingredients:

- 1 cup uncooked quinoa
- 1 lb ground turkey
- 1 tbsp sesame oil
- 2 cups mixed vegetables
(such as broccoli, bell peppers,
snap peas, carrots)

- 2 tbsp low-sodium soy sauce
- 1 tbsp rice vinegar
- 2 cloves garlic, minced
- 1 tbsp grated fresh ginger
- 1 tsp honey
- 1/4 tsp red pepper flakes (optional)
- Salt and pepper to taste
- 2 tbsp chopped green onions (for garnish)

Instructions:

1. Cook the quinoa according to package instructions. Set aside.

2. In a large skillet or wok, cook the ground turkey over medium-high heat, breaking it up with a wooden spoon, until browned and cooked through, about 5-7 minutes. Remove the turkey from the pan and set aside.

3. In the same pan, heat the sesame oil over high heat. Add the mixed vegetables and stir-fry for 3-4 minutes, until they are tender-crisp.

4. Add the garlic and ginger to the pan and cook for 1 minute, until fragrant.

5. Return the cooked turkey to the pan. Stir in the soy sauce, rice vinegar, honey, and red pepper flakes (if using). Season with salt and pepper to taste.

6. Cook the stir-fry for an additional 2-3 minutes, until everything is heated through.

7. Serve the turkey and vegetable stir-fry over the cooked quinoa, garnished with chopped green onions.

This recipe is an excellent choice for athletes for several reasons:

- Ground turkey is a lean protein source to support muscle recovery and growth.
- Quinoa is a complete protein that also provides complex carbohydrates to fuel your workouts.
- The variety of vegetables (broccoli, bell peppers, snap peas, carrots) offer a range of vitamins, minerals, and antioxidants.
- The stir-fry is flavored with garlic, ginger, soy sauce, and rice vinegar, adding flavor without excessive sodium or sugar.

This dish is well-balanced, nutrient-dense, and can be easily customized with your favorite vegetables or protein sources. Enjoy this turkey and vegetable stir-fry with quinoa as part of a healthy, athlete-friendly diet.

25. Greek yogurt chicken salad with grapes and walnuts

Ingredients:
- 2 cups cooked, shredded chicken breast
- 1 cup plain Greek yogurt
- 1/2 cup halved red grapes
- 1/4 cup chopped walnuts
- 2 tbsp chopped fresh parsley
- 1 tbsp lemon juice
- 1/4 tsp salt
- 1/4 tsp black pepper

Instructions:

1. In a large bowl, combine the shredded chicken, Greek yogurt, grapes, walnuts, parsley, lemon juice, salt, and pepper. Stir until well mixed.

2. Serve the chicken salad on a bed of greens, in a whole wheat pita, or on top of crackers.

This recipe is perfect for athletes as it provides a good balance of protein from the chicken, healthy fats from the walnuts, and carbohydrates from the grapes. The Greek yogurt adds creaminess and extra protein. It's a nutritious and satisfying meal or snack.

26. Black bean and vegetable quesadillas
with whole wheat tortillas

Ingredients:
- 1 (15 oz) can black beans, rinsed and drained
- 1 cup diced bell peppers (any color)
- 1/2 cup diced onion
- 1 cup shredded low-fat cheddar or Monterey Jack cheese
- 8 whole wheat tortillas
- 1 tbsp olive oil
- Salt and pepper to taste

Instructions:

1. In a medium bowl, mash the black beans slightly with a fork or potato masher. Stir in the diced bell peppers and onions.

2. Lay 4 of the whole wheat tortillas on a flat surface. Divide the black bean mixture evenly among the tortillas, spreading it to the edges. Sprinkle the shredded cheese on top.

3. Place the remaining 4 tortillas on top to make quesadillas.

4. Heat the olive oil in a large skillet over medium heat. Cook the quesadillas in batches for 2-3 minutes per side, until the tortillas are lightly browned and the cheese is melted.

5. Cut each quesadilla into wedges and serve warm.

These quesadillas are perfect for athletes as they provide complex carbs from the whole wheat tortillas, fiber and protein from the black beans, and nutrients from the vegetables. The cheese adds calcium and protein as well. Enjoy!

27. Baked falafel with tabbouleh and hummus

Falafel Ingredients:
- 1 (15 oz) can chickpeas, rinsed and drained
- 1/2 cup chopped parsley
- 1/4 cup chopped cilantro
- 2 cloves garlic, minced
- 1 tsp ground cumin
- 1/2 tsp ground coriander
- 1/4 tsp cayenne pepper
- 2 tbsp whole wheat flour
- Salt and pepper to taste

Tabbouleh Ingredients:
- 1 cup bulgur wheat
- 1 cup chopped parsley
- 1/2 cup chopped tomatoes
- 1/4 cup chopped mint
- 2 tbsp lemon juice
- 1 tbsp olive oil
- Salt and pepper to taste

To Serve:
- 1 cup hummus
- Whole wheat pita bread or lettuce leaves

Instructions:

1. Preheat oven to 400°F. Line a baking sheet with parchment paper.

2. Make the falafel: In a food processor, pulse the chickpeas, parsley, cilantro, garlic, cumin, coriander, and cayenne until coarsely chopped. Transfer to a bowl and stir in the flour, salt, and pepper. Form into 12 small patties.

3. Arrange the falafel patties on the prepared baking sheet. Bake for 15-20 minutes, flipping halfway, until golden brown.

4. Make the tabbouleh: In a medium bowl, combine the bulgur, parsley, tomatoes, mint, lemon juice, and olive oil. Season with salt and pepper.

5. Serve the baked falafel with the tabbouleh salad and hummus, with pita bread or lettuce leaves on the side.

This meal is perfect for athletes as it provides complex carbs, protein, fiber, and healthy fats from the chickpeas, bulgur, and olive oil. The herbs and vegetables also pack in important vitamins and minerals.

28. Grilled vegetable and quinoa salad with balsamic vinaigrette

Salad Ingredients:
- 1 cup uncooked quinoa, rinsed
- 2 cups vegetable or chicken broth
- 1 zucchini, sliced into 1/2-inch rounds
- 1 yellow squash, sliced into 1/2-inch rounds
- 1 red bell pepper, cut into 1-inch pieces
- 1 red onion, sliced into 1/2-inch rounds
- 2 cups baby spinach
- 1/4 cup crumbled feta cheese (optional)

Balsamic Vinaigrette:
- 3 tbsp balsamic vinegar
- 2 tbsp olive oil
- 1 tbsp Dijon mustard
- 1 tsp honey
- 1 garlic clove, minced
- Salt and pepper to taste

Instructions:

1. Cook the quinoa according to package instructions using the broth instead of water. Fluff with a fork and set aside to cool.

2. Preheat grill or grill pan to medium-high heat. Grill the zucchini, squash, bell pepper, and onion slices for 2-3 minutes per side until charred and tender.

3. In a large bowl, combine the grilled vegetables, cooked quinoa, and spinach.

4. In a small bowl, whisk together the vinaigrette ingredients.

5. Drizzle the vinaigrette over the salad and toss to coat. Top with crumbled feta if desired.

6. Serve immediately or refrigerate until ready to serve.

This salad is perfect for athletes as it's packed with complex carbs from the quinoa, fiber and vitamins from the vegetables, and healthy fats from the olive oil. The balsamic vinaigrette adds flavor without too many calories. Enjoy!

29. Turkey and barley soup with mixed vegetables

Ingredients:
- 1 lb ground turkey
- 1 onion, diced
- 3 carrots, peeled and diced
- 3 celery stalks, diced
- 3 garlic cloves, minced
- 8 cups low-sodium chicken or vegetable broth
- 1 cup pearl barley, rinsed
- 1 (15 oz) can diced tomatoes
- 2 cups frozen mixed vegetables (peas, corn, green beans)
- 2 tsp dried thyme
- 1 tsp dried oregano
- Salt and pepper to taste

Instructions:

1. In a large pot or Dutch oven, cook the ground turkey over medium-high heat, breaking it up with a wooden spoon, until browned, about 5-7 minutes. Drain any excess fat.

2. Add the onion, carrots, celery, and garlic to the pot. Cook for 5 minutes, stirring occasionally, until the vegetables start to soften.

3. Pour in the broth and add the barley. Bring to a boil, then reduce heat and simmer for 25-30 minutes, until the barley is tender.

4. Stir in the diced tomatoes, frozen mixed vegetables, thyme, and oregano. Season with salt and pepper to taste.

5. Simmer for an additional 10-15 minutes, until the vegetables are heated through.

6. Serve the soup hot. Garnish with extra herbs if desired.

This soup is perfect for athletes as it provides complex carbs from the barley, lean protein from the turkey, and a variety of vitamins and minerals from the vegetables. The broth keeps it hydrating as well. Enjoy!

30. Lemon herb grilled chicken
with roasted asparagus and cauliflower rice

Ingredients:
Chicken:
- 4 boneless, skinless chicken breasts
- 2 tbsp olive oil
- 2 tbsp lemon juice
- 1 tbsp chopped fresh parsley
- 1 tbsp chopped fresh thyme
- 1 tsp garlic powder
- Salt and pepper to taste

Asparagus:
- 1 lb asparagus, trimmed
- 1 tbsp olive oil
- Salt and pepper to taste

Cauliflower Rice:
- 1 head cauliflower, grated or pulsed in a food processor
- 1 tbsp olive oil
- Salt and pepper to taste

Instructions:
1. Preheat grill or grill pan to medium-high heat.

2. In a shallow dish, combine the olive oil, lemon juice, parsley, thyme, garlic powder, salt and pepper. Add the chicken breasts and turn to coat both sides.

3. Grill the chicken for 5-7 minutes per side, until cooked through.

4. Toss the asparagus with olive oil, salt and pepper. Spread on a baking sheet and roast at 400°F for 12-15 minutes, until tender.

5. In a large skillet, heat the olive oil over medium heat. Add the grated cauliflower and sauté for 5-7 minutes, until tender. Season with salt and pepper.

6. Serve the grilled chicken with the roasted asparagus and cauliflower rice. Enjoy!

This meal is perfect for athletes as it provides lean protein from the chicken, complex carbs from the cauliflower rice, and fiber and nutrients from the asparagus. The lemon and herbs add great flavor without extra calories. It's a balanced, nutrient-dense dish.

31. Asian-style tofu and vegetable stir-fry with brown rice

Ingredients:
Stir-Fry:
- 1 block extra-firm tofu, cubed
- 2 tbsp sesame oil
- 2 cups mixed vegetables (broccoli, bell peppers, snap peas, etc.)
- 3 cloves garlic, minced
- 1 tbsp grated fresh ginger
- 2 tbsp low-sodium soy sauce
- 1 tbsp rice vinegar
- 1 tsp honey
- 1/4 tsp red pepper flakes (optional)
- Salt and pepper to taste

Brown Rice:
- 1 cup uncooked brown rice
- 2 cups low-sodium vegetable or chicken broth

Instructions:

1. Cook the brown rice: In a medium saucepan, bring the broth to a boil. Add the rice, cover, and reduce heat to low. Simmer for 25-30 minutes until rice is tender. Fluff with a fork.

2. Make the stir-fry: In a large skillet or wok, heat the sesame oil over medium-high heat. Add the tofu cubes and cook for 2-3 minutes per side until lightly browned.

3. Add the mixed vegetables, garlic, and ginger to the pan. Stir-fry for 5-7 minutes until vegetables are tender-crisp.

4. In a small bowl, whisk together the soy sauce, rice vinegar, and honey. Pour the sauce into the pan and toss to coat everything evenly.

5. If using, sprinkle in the red pepper flakes. Season with salt and pepper to taste.

6. Serve the stir-fried tofu and vegetables over the cooked brown rice.

This dish is perfect for athletes as it provides plant-based protein from the tofu, complex carbs from the brown rice, and a variety of vitamins and minerals from the vegetables. The ginger, garlic, and soy sauce add great Asian-inspired flavor.

32. Lentil and vegetable curry with quinoa

Ingredients:
Curry:
- 1 cup dry red lentils, rinsed
- 1 tbsp olive oil
- 1 onion, diced
- 3 cloves garlic, minced
- 1 tbsp grated fresh ginger
- 2 tsp garam masala
- 1 tsp ground cumin
- 1 tsp ground coriander
- 1 (14 oz) can diced tomatoes
- 1 (13.5 oz) can coconut milk
- 2 cups mixed vegetables (cauliflower, potatoes, spinach, etc.)
- Salt and pepper to taste

Quinoa:
- 1 cup uncooked quinoa, rinsed
- 2 cups low-sodium vegetable or chicken broth

Instructions:
1. Cook the quinoa: In a medium saucepan, bring the broth to a boil. Add the quinoa, cover, and reduce heat to low. Simmer for 15-20 minutes until quinoa is tender. Fluff with a fork.

2. Make the curry: In a large pot or Dutch oven, heat the olive oil over medium heat. Add the onion and sauté for 5 minutes until translucent.

3. Stir in the garlic, ginger, garam masala, cumin, and coriander. Cook for 1 minute until fragrant.

4. Add the lentils, diced tomatoes, coconut milk, and mixed vegetables. Bring to a simmer and cook for 20-25 minutes, until lentils are tender and vegetables are cooked through.

5. Season the curry with salt and pepper to taste.

6. Serve the lentil curry over the cooked quinoa. Garnish with fresh cilantro if desired.

This curry dish is perfect for athletes as it provides plant-based protein from the lentils, complex carbs from the quinoa, and a variety of nutrients from the vegetables. The coconut milk adds creaminess and healthy fats. Enjoy!

33. Baked halibut with roasted root vegetables

Ingredients:
Roasted Vegetables:
- 2 cups cubed sweet potatoes
- 2 cups cubed beet
- 1 cup cubed parsnips
- 1 cup cubed carrots
- 2 tbsp olive oil
- Salt and pepper to taste

Halibut:
- 4 (6 oz) halibut fillets
- 2 tbsp olive oil
- 1 tsp lemon zest
- 2 tbsp chopped fresh parsley
- Salt and pepper to taste

Instructions:

1. Preheat oven to 400°F. Line a large baking sheet with parchment paper.

2. In a large bowl, toss the cubed root vegetables with the olive oil, salt, and pepper. Spread in a single layer on the prepared baking sheet.

3. Roast the vegetables for 25-30 minutes, stirring halfway, until tender and lightly browned.

4. Meanwhile, place the halibut fillets on a separate baking sheet. Drizzle with olive oil and sprinkle with lemon zest, parsley, salt, and pepper.

5. Bake the halibut for 12-15 minutes, until it flakes easily with a fork.

6. Serve the baked halibut fillets with the roasted root vegetables. Garnish with extra parsley if desired.

This meal is perfect for athletes as it provides lean protein from the halibut, complex carbs from the root vegetables, and healthy fats from the olive oil. The vegetables also provide important vitamins, minerals, and antioxidants. It's a nutrient-dense and satisfying dish.

34. Whole wheat pita pizzas with chicken, spinach, and tomatoes

Ingredients:
- 4 whole wheat pita breads
- 1 cup shredded cooked chicken breast
- 1 cup baby spinach leaves
- 1 cup diced tomatoes
- 1 cup shredded part-skim mozzarella cheese
- 2 tbsp olive oil
- 1 tsp dried oregano
- Salt and pepper to taste

Instructions:

1. Preheat oven to 400°F. Line a baking sheet with parchment paper.

2. Place the whole wheat pita breads on the prepared baking sheet.

3. In a bowl, mix together the shredded chicken, spinach, tomatoes, and mozzarella cheese.

4. Drizzle the pita breads with the olive oil and sprinkle with the dried oregano, salt, and pepper.

5. Divide the chicken and vegetable mixture evenly among the pita breads, spreading it to the edges.

6. Bake for 10-12 minutes, until the cheese is melted and the pita is lightly golden.

7. Slice each pita pizza into quarters and serve immediately.

These whole wheat pita pizzas are perfect for athletes as they provide a balance of lean protein from the chicken, complex carbs from the whole wheat pita, and fiber and nutrients from the spinach and tomatoes. The mozzarella cheese adds calcium. It's a quick, easy, and nutritious meal.

35. Shrimp and vegetable stir-fry with soba noodles

Ingredients:
- 8 oz soba noodles
- 1 lb shrimp, peeled and deveined
- 2 tbsp sesame oil, divided
- 2 cups mixed vegetables (broccoli, bell peppers, snap peas, etc.)
- 3 cloves garlic, minced
- 1 tbsp grated fresh ginger
- 2 tbsp low-sodium soy sauce
- 1 tbsp rice vinegar
- 1 tsp honey
- Salt and pepper to taste
- Chopped green onions for garnish (optional)

Instructions:
1. Cook the soba noodles according to package instructions. Drain and rinse under cold water. Set aside.

2. In a large skillet or wok, heat 1 tbsp of the sesame oil over medium-high heat. Add the shrimp and stir-fry for 2-3 minutes until opaque. Remove shrimp from pan and set aside.

3. Add the remaining 1 tbsp of sesame oil to the pan. Stir-fry the mixed vegetables for 4-5 minutes until tender-crisp.

4. Add the garlic and ginger to the pan and cook for 1 minute until fragrant.

5. Return the cooked shrimp to the pan. Add the soy sauce, rice vinegar, and honey. Toss to coat everything evenly.

6. Add the cooked soba noodles and toss the entire stir-fry together until well combined and heated through.

7. Season with salt and pepper to taste.

8. Serve the shrimp and vegetable stir-fry with soba noodles, garnished with chopped green onions if desired.

This dish is perfect for athletes as it provides lean protein from the shrimp, complex carbs from the soba noodles, and a variety of vitamins and minerals from the vegetables. The ginger, garlic, and soy sauce add great Asian-inspired flavor.

36. Greek turkey meatloaf with mashed sweet potatoes

Meatloaf Ingredients:
- 1 lb ground turkey
- 1/2 cup crumbled feta cheese
- 1/2 cup chopped fresh parsley
- 1/4 cup panko breadcrumbs
- 2 cloves garlic, minced
- 1 tsp dried oregano
- 1/2 tsp ground cinnamon
- 1/4 tsp red pepper flakes (optional)
- Salt and pepper to taste

Mashed Sweet Potatoes:
- 3 medium sweet potatoes, peeled and cubed
- 2 tbsp unsweetened almond milk
- 1 tbsp olive oil
- 1 tsp ground cinnamon
- Salt and pepper to taste

Instructions:

1. Preheat oven to 375°F. Lightly grease a 9x5 inch loaf pan.

2. In a large bowl, combine all the meatloaf ingredients until well mixed. Transfer the mixture to the prepared loaf pan, packing it down firmly.

3. Bake the meatloaf for 45-55 minutes, until cooked through. Let rest for 5 minutes before slicing.

4. While the meatloaf is baking, place the cubed sweet potatoes in a pot and cover with water. Bring to a boil and cook for 15-20 minutes until very soft.

5. Drain the sweet potatoes and return to the pot. Mash with the almond milk, olive oil, cinnamon, salt and pepper until smooth and creamy.

6. Serve slices of the Greek turkey meatloaf with the mashed sweet potatoes on the side.

This meal is perfect for athletes as it provides lean protein from the turkey, complex carbs from the sweet potatoes, and healthy fats from the olive oil. The feta, herbs, and spices add great Mediterranean flavor. It's a nutritious and satisfying dish.

37. Quinoa and black bean stuffed bell peppers

Ingredients:
- 4 large bell peppers, halved lengthwise and seeds removed
- 1 cup cooked quinoa
- 1 (15 oz) can black beans, rinsed and drained
- 1 cup diced tomatoes
- 1/2 cup crumbled feta cheese
- 1/4 cup chopped fresh cilantro
- 2 cloves garlic, minced
- 1 tsp ground cumin
- 1/2 tsp chili powder
- Salt and pepper to taste

Instructions:

1. Preheat oven to 375°F. Arrange the bell pepper halves in a baking dish.

2. In a large bowl, combine the cooked quinoa, black beans, diced tomatoes, feta cheese, cilantro, garlic, cumin, chili powder, salt, and pepper. Stir until well mixed.

3. Spoon the quinoa and black bean mixture evenly into the bell pepper halves, packing it in gently.

4. Cover the baking dish with foil and bake for 30 minutes.

5. Remove the foil and bake for an additional 10-15 minutes, until the peppers are tender and the filling is hot.

6. Serve the stuffed bell peppers warm.

This dish is perfect for athletes as it provides complex carbs from the quinoa, fiber and protein from the black beans, and a variety of vitamins and minerals from the bell peppers and other vegetables. The feta cheese adds calcium. It's a well-balanced and nutrient-dense meal.

38. Baked chicken drumsticks with roasted carrots and parsnips

Ingredients:
Chicken:
- 8 chicken drumsticks
- 2 tbsp olive oil
- 1 tsp paprika
- 1 tsp garlic powder
- 1/2 tsp dried thyme
- Salt and pepper to taste

Roasted Vegetables:
- 3 carrots, peeled and cut into 1-inch pieces
- 3 parsnips, peeled and cut into 1-inch pieces
- 2 tbsp olive oil
- 1 tsp dried rosemary
- Salt and pepper to taste

Instructions:

1. Preheat oven to 400°F. Line a large baking sheet with parchment paper.

2. In a large bowl, toss the chicken drumsticks with the olive oil, paprika, garlic powder, thyme, salt, and pepper until evenly coated.

3. Arrange the chicken drumsticks on one side of the prepared baking sheet.

4. In the same bowl, toss the carrot and parsnip pieces with the olive oil, rosemary, salt, and pepper.

5. Spread the seasoned vegetables on the other side of the baking sheet, making sure they are in a single layer.

6. Bake for 35-40 minutes, flipping the chicken and stirring the vegetables halfway, until the chicken is cooked through and the vegetables are tender.

7. Serve the baked chicken drumsticks with the roasted carrots and parsnips.

This meal is perfect for athletes as it provides lean protein from the chicken, complex carbs from the root vegetables, and a variety of vitamins and minerals. The simple seasoning allows the natural flavors to shine. It's a nutritious and satisfying dish.

39. Tuna salad lettuce wraps with avocado and tomatoes

Ingredients:
- 2 (5 oz) cans tuna, drained and flaked
- 1/4 cup plain Greek yogurt
- 1 tbsp Dijon mustard
- 1 tbsp lemon juice
- 2 tbsp finely chopped celery
- 2 tbsp finely chopped red onion
- 2 tbsp chopped fresh parsley
- Salt and pepper to taste
- 4-6 large lettuce leaves (such as romaine or butter lettuce)
- 1 avocado, sliced
- 1 cup cherry tomatoes, halved

Instructions:

1. In a medium bowl, combine the tuna, Greek yogurt, Dijon mustard, lemon juice, celery, red onion, and parsley. Mix well and season with salt and pepper.

2. Lay the lettuce leaves flat on a plate or work surface. Divide the tuna salad evenly among the lettuce leaves.

3. Top each tuna salad-filled lettuce wrap with sliced avocado and halved cherry tomatoes.

4. Serve the tuna salad lettuce wraps immediately.

This recipe is perfect for athletes as it provides lean protein from the tuna, healthy fats from the avocado, and a variety of vitamins and minerals from the vegetables. The Greek yogurt adds creaminess without too many calories. It's a light, refreshing, and nutrient-dense meal.

You can adjust the amounts of each ingredient to suit your preferences or the number of servings needed. Enjoy!

40. Veggie-packed turkey and bean chili

Ingredients:
- 1 lb ground turkey
- 1 tbsp olive oil
- 1 onion, diced
- 3 cloves garlic, minced
- 2 bell peppers, diced
- 2 carrots, peeled and diced
- 2 celery stalks, diced
- 1 (15 oz) can black beans, rinsed and drained
- 1 (15 oz) can kidney beans, rinsed and drained
- 1 (28 oz) can diced tomatoes
- 2 tbsp chili powder
- 1 tsp ground cumin
- 1 tsp dried oregano
- 1/2 tsp smoked paprika
- Salt and pepper to taste
- Chopped cilantro for garnish (optional)

Instructions:

1. In a large pot or Dutch oven, cook the ground turkey over medium-high heat, breaking it up with a wooden spoon, until browned, about 5-7 minutes. Drain any excess fat.

2. Add the olive oil to the pot. Sauté the onion, garlic, bell peppers, carrots, and celery for 5-7 minutes until softened.

3. Stir in the black beans, kidney beans, diced tomatoes, chili powder, cumin, oregano, and smoked paprika. Season with salt and pepper.

4. Bring the chili to a simmer and let it cook for 20-25 minutes, stirring occasionally, until thickened.

5. Serve the turkey and bean chili hot, garnished with chopped cilantro if desired. Can be served over brown rice or quinoa.

This chili is perfect for athletes as it provides lean protein from the turkey, fiber and complex carbs from the beans and vegetables, and a variety of vitamins and minerals. The spices add great flavor without too many calories. It's a hearty and nutritious meal.

41. Grilled swordfish with quinoa salad and grilled zucchini

Ingredients:
Swordfish:
- 4 (6 oz) swordfish steaks
- 2 tbsp olive oil
- 1 tsp lemon zest
- Salt and pepper to taste

Grilled Zucchini:
- 2 medium zucchini, sliced lengthwise into 1/2-inch thick strips
- 1 tbsp olive oil
- Salt and pepper to taste

Quinoa Salad:
- 1 cup uncooked quinoa, rinsed
- 1 cup cherry tomatoes, halved
- 1/2 cup diced cucumber
- 1/4 cup crumbled feta cheese
- 2 tbsp chopped fresh parsley
- 2 tbsp lemon juice
- 1 tbsp olive oil
- Salt and pepper to taste

Instructions:

1. Preheat grill or grill pan to medium-high heat.

2. Prepare the swordfish: Brush the swordfish steaks with olive oil and season with lemon zest, salt, and pepper.

3. Grill the swordfish for 4-5 minutes per side, until cooked through and opaque.

4. Make the quinoa salad: Cook the quinoa according to package instructions. Fluff with a fork and let cool slightly.

5. In a bowl, combine the cooked quinoa, cherry tomatoes, cucumber, feta, parsley, lemon juice, and olive oil. Season with salt and pepper.

6. Prepare the grilled zucchini: Brush the zucchini strips with olive oil and season with salt and pepper.

7. Grill the zucchini for 2-3 minutes per side, until tender and charred.

8. Serve the grilled swordfish with the quinoa salad and grilled zucchini on the side.

This meal is perfect for athletes as it provides lean protein from the swordfish, complex carbs from the quinoa, and a variety of vitamins and minerals from the vegetables. The healthy fats from the olive oil and quinoa also make this a well-balanced and nutrient-dense dish.

42. Moroccan chickpea stew with couscous

Ingredients:

Stew:
- 2 tbsp olive oil
- 1 onion, diced
- 3 cloves garlic, minced
- 1 tbsp grated fresh ginger
- 2 tsp ground cumin
- 1 tsp ground coriander

Couscous:
- 1 cup uncooked whole wheat couscous
- 1 cup low-sodium vegetable or chicken broth

- 1 tsp paprika
- 1/4 tsp cayenne pepper (optional)
- 1 (15 oz) can chickpeas, rinsed and drained
- 1 (14 oz) can diced tomatoes
- 1 cup low-sodium vegetable or chicken broth
- 1 cup diced sweet potatoes
- 1 cup frozen peas
- Salt and pepper to taste
- Chopped cilantro for garnish

Instructions:

1. In a large pot or Dutch oven, heat the olive oil over medium heat. Add the onion and sauté for 5 minutes until translucent.

2. Stir in the garlic, ginger, cumin, coriander, paprika, and cayenne (if using). Cook for 1 minute until fragrant.

3. Add the chickpeas, diced tomatoes, broth, sweet potatoes, and peas. Season with salt and pepper.

4. Bring the stew to a simmer and cook for 20-25 minutes, until the sweet potatoes are tender.

5. Meanwhile, prepare the couscous: In a medium saucepan, bring the broth to a boil. Remove from heat, stir in the couscous, cover and let stand for 5 minutes. Fluff with a fork.

6. Serve the Moroccan chickpea stew over the cooked couscous, garnished with chopped cilantro.

This dish is perfect for athletes as it provides plant-based protein from the chickpeas, complex carbs from the couscous and sweet potatoes, and a variety of vitamins and minerals from the vegetables. The Moroccan spices add great flavor without too many calories.

43. Turkey sausage and vegetable frittata

Ingredients:
- 8 eggs
- 1/4 cup unsweetened almond milk
- 1/4 tsp salt
- 1/4 tsp black pepper
- 1 tbsp olive oil
- 3 links turkey sausage, casings removed and crumbled
- 1 cup diced bell peppers
- 1 cup diced onions
- 2 cups baby spinach, chopped
- 1/2 cup shredded cheddar cheese

Instructions:

1. Preheat oven to 375°F. Grease a 9-inch pie dish or oven-safe skillet.

2. In a large bowl, whisk together the eggs, almond milk, salt, and pepper until well combined.

3. In a skillet over medium heat, cook the crumbled turkey sausage until browned, 5-7 minutes. Remove sausage from pan and set aside.

4. Add the olive oil to the same skillet. Sauté the bell peppers and onions for 5 minutes until softened.

5. Add the spinach to the skillet and cook for 1-2 minutes until wilted.

6. Pour the egg mixture into the prepared pie dish or skillet. Top evenly with the cooked sausage, vegetables, and shredded cheese.

7. Bake for 20-25 minutes, until the center is set and the edges are lightly golden.

8. Let the frittata cool for 5 minutes before slicing and serving.

This frittata is perfect for athletes as it provides lean protein from the turkey sausage, vegetables for fiber and nutrients, and eggs for additional protein. The cheese adds calcium. It's a nutrient-dense and satisfying meal.

You can customize the vegetables based on your preferences. Enjoy!

44. Baked tofu with sesame ginger sauce and steamed broccoli

Ingredients:
Tofu:
- 1 block (14 oz) extra-firm tofu, pressed and cubed
- 1 tbsp sesame oil
- 1 tbsp low-sodium soy sauce

Sesame Ginger Sauce:
- 2 tbsp low-sodium soy sauce
- 1 tbsp rice vinegar
- 1 tbsp honey
- 1 tsp sesame oil
- 1 tsp grated fresh ginger
- 1 clove garlic, minced
- 1/4 tsp red pepper flakes (optional)

Broccoli:
- 4 cups broccoli florets
- 1 tbsp water

Instructions:

1. Preheat oven to 400°F. Line a baking sheet with parchment paper.

2. In a bowl, toss the cubed tofu with the 1 tbsp sesame oil and 1 tbsp soy sauce until evenly coated. Spread the tofu on the prepared baking sheet.

3. Bake the tofu for 20-25 minutes, flipping halfway, until golden brown.

4. Meanwhile, make the sesame ginger sauce: In a small bowl, whisk together the 2 tbsp soy sauce, rice vinegar, honey, 1 tsp sesame oil, ginger, garlic, and red pepper flakes (if using).

5. In a steamer basket, steam the broccoli florets with the 1 tbsp water for 5-7 minutes until tender-crisp.

6. Serve the baked tofu drizzled with the sesame ginger sauce, alongside the steamed broccoli.

This meal is perfect for athletes as it provides plant-based protein from the tofu, complex carbs from the broccoli, and healthy fats from the sesame oil. The ginger and garlic add great flavor without extra calories. It's a nutritious and satisfying dish.

45. Greek-style grilled shrimp with orzo and roasted vegetables

Ingredients:
Shrimp:
- 1 lb large shrimp, peeled and deveined
- 2 tbsp olive oil
- 2 tbsp lemon juice
- 1 tsp dried oregano
- 1/2 tsp garlic powder
- Salt and pepper to taste

Orzo:
- 1 cup uncooked orzo pasta
- 2 cups low-sodium chicken or vegetable broth

Roasted Vegetables:
- 2 cups cubed zucchini
- 2 cups cubed eggplant
- 1 red onion, sliced
- 2 tbsp olive oil
- 1 tsp dried oregano
- Salt and pepper to taste

Instructions:

1. Preheat grill or grill pan to medium-high heat.

2. In a bowl, toss the shrimp with the 2 tbsp olive oil, lemon juice, 1 tsp oregano, garlic powder, salt, and pepper.

3. Thread the seasoned shrimp onto skewers.

4. Grill the shrimp skewers for 2-3 minutes per side, until opaque and cooked through.

5. Meanwhile, cook the orzo: In a saucepan, bring the broth to a boil. Add the orzo, cover, and reduce heat to low. Simmer for 12-15 minutes until tender. Drain and fluff with a fork.

6. Roast the vegetables: Preheat oven to 400°F. On a baking sheet, toss the zucchini, eggplant, and onion with the 2 tbsp olive oil, 1 tsp oregano, salt, and pepper. Roast for 20-25 minutes, stirring halfway, until tender.

7. Serve the grilled shrimp over the cooked orzo, topped with the roasted vegetables.

This meal is perfect for athletes as it provides lean protein from the shrimp, complex carbs from the orzo, and a variety of vitamins and minerals from the roasted vegetables. The Greek-inspired flavors make it a delicious and nutritious option.

46. Chicken and vegetable curry with brown rice

Ingredients:
Curry:
- 1 lb boneless, skinless chicken breasts, cubed
- 2 tbsp olive oil
- 1 onion, diced
- 3 cloves garlic, minced
- 1 tbsp grated fresh ginger
- 2 tsp curry powder
- 1 tsp ground cumin
- 1 tsp ground coriander
- 1 (14 oz) can diced tomatoes
- 1 (13.5 oz) can coconut milk
- 2 cups mixed vegetables (cauliflower, potatoes, spinach, etc.)
- Salt and pepper to taste

Brown Rice:
- 1 cup uncooked brown rice
- 2 cups low-sodium chicken or vegetable broth

Instructions:
1. Cook the brown rice: In a medium saucepan, bring the broth to a boil. Add the rice, cover, and reduce heat to low. Simmer for 25-30 minutes until rice is tender. Fluff with a fork.

2. Make the curry: In a large skillet or Dutch oven, heat the olive oil over medium heat. Add the chicken and sauté for 5-7 minutes until lightly browned.

3. Add the onion, garlic, and ginger to the pan. Cook for 2-3 minutes until fragrant.

4. Stir in the curry powder, cumin, and coriander. Cook for 1 minute.

5. Pour in the diced tomatoes and coconut milk. Add the mixed vegetables and season with salt and pepper.

6. Bring the curry to a simmer and cook for 15-20 minutes, until the chicken is cooked through and the vegetables are tender. Serve the chicken and vegetable curry over the cooked brown rice.

This curry dish is perfect for athletes as it provides lean protein from the chicken, complex carbs from the brown rice, and a variety of nutrients from the vegetables. The coconut milk adds creaminess and healthy fats. It's a well-balanced and flavorful meal.

47. Lentil and vegetable shepherd's pie with mashed cauliflower topping

Ingredients:

Filling:

- 1 cup dry brown or green lentils, rinsed
- 3 cups low-sodium vegetable broth
- 1 tbsp olive oil
- 1 onion, diced
- 3 carrots, peeled and diced
- 2 celery stalks, diced
- 3 cloves garlic, minced
- 1 tsp dried thyme
- 1 tsp dried rosemary
- 1 (15 oz) can diced tomatoes
- Salt and pepper to taste

Mashed Cauliflower Topping:

- 1 head cauliflower, cut into florets
- 2 tbsp unsweetened almond milk
- 2 tbsp grated Parmesan cheese
- Salt and pepper to taste

Instructions:

1. Preheat oven to 375°F. Grease a 9x13 inch baking dish.

2. In a saucepan, combine the lentils and vegetable broth. Bring to a boil, then reduce heat and simmer for 20-25 minutes until lentils are tender. Drain any excess liquid.

3. In a large skillet, heat the olive oil over medium heat. Add the onion, carrots, celery, and garlic. Sauté for 5-7 minutes until vegetables are softened.

4. Stir the cooked lentils, diced tomatoes, thyme, and rosemary into the vegetable mixture. Season with salt and pepper.

5. Spread the lentil and vegetable filling into the prepared baking dish.

6. Make the mashed cauliflower topping: In a large pot, cover the cauliflower florets with water and bring to a boil. Cook for 10-12 minutes until very tender. Drain and return to the pot.

7. Mash the cauliflower with the almond milk and Parmesan. Season with salt and pepper.

8. Spread the mashed cauliflower evenly over the lentil filling. Bake the shepherd's pie for 25-30 minutes, until the topping is lightly browned. Let stand for 5 minutes before serving.

This shepherd's pie is perfect for athletes as it provides plant-based protein from the lentils, complex carbs from the cauliflower, and a variety of nutrients from the vegetables. It's a hearty and satisfying meal.

48. Black bean and corn salad with avocado and lime dressing

Ingredients:
Salad:
- 1 (15 oz) can black beans, rinsed and drained
- 1 cup frozen corn, thawed
- 1 cup diced tomatoes
- 1/2 cup diced red onion
- 1/4 cup chopped fresh cilantro

Dressing:
- 1 avocado, pitted and mashed
- 2 tbsp lime juice
- 1 tbsp olive oil
- 1 tsp honey
- 1 garlic clove, minced
- Salt and pepper to taste

Instructions:

1. In a large bowl, combine the black beans, corn, tomatoes, red onion, and cilantro. Toss to mix.

2. In a small bowl, whisk together the mashed avocado, lime juice, olive oil, honey, and garlic. Season with salt and pepper.

3. Pour the avocado lime dressing over the black bean and corn salad. Toss gently to coat.

4. Refrigerate the salad for at least 30 minutes to allow the flavors to meld.

5. Serve chilled or at room temperature.

This black bean and corn salad is perfect for athletes as it provides plant-based protein from the black beans, complex carbs from the corn, and healthy fats from the avocado. The lime dressing adds a refreshing zing. It's a nutritious and flavorful dish.

You can adjust the amounts of each ingredient to suit your preferences or the number of servings needed. Enjoy!

49. Teriyaki chicken and vegetable skewers with brown rice

Ingredients:
***Skewers*:**

- 1 lb boneless, skinless chicken breasts,
cut into 1-inch cubes
- 1 red bell pepper, cut into 1-inch pieces
- 1 yellow bell pepper, cut into 1-inch pieces
- 1 red onion, cut into 1-inch pieces
- 8 oz mushrooms, halved

Teriyaki Sauce:

- 1/2 cup low-sodium soy sauce
- 2 tbsp honey
- 2 tbsp rice vinegar
- 1 tbsp sesame oil
- 2 cloves garlic, minced
- 1 tsp grated fresh ginger

Brown Rice:

- 1 cup uncooked brown rice
- 2 cups low-sodium chicken or vegetable broth

Instructions:

1. Make the teriyaki sauce: In a small bowl, whisk together the soy sauce, honey, rice vinegar, sesame oil, garlic, and ginger. Set aside.

2. Cook the brown rice: In a medium saucepan, bring the broth to a boil. Add the rice, cover, and reduce heat to low. Simmer for 25-30 minutes until rice is tender. Fluff with a fork.

3. Thread the chicken and vegetables onto skewers, alternating the ingredients.

4. Preheat grill or grill pan to medium-high heat.

5. Grill the skewers for 8-10 minutes, turning occasionally, until the chicken is cooked through.

6. Brush the skewers generously with the teriyaki sauce during the last 2-3 minutes of cooking. Serve the grilled chicken and vegetable skewers over the cooked brown rice.

This meal is perfect for athletes as it provides lean protein from the chicken, complex carbs from the brown rice, and a variety of vitamins and minerals from the vegetables. The teriyaki sauce adds great flavor without too many calories. It's a well-balanced and satisfying dish.

50. Quinoa and vegetable stuffed portobello mushrooms

Ingredients:
- 4 large portobello mushroom caps, stems removed and chopped
- 1 cup cooked quinoa
- 1 cup diced bell peppers
- 1/2 cup diced onion
- 1/2 cup diced zucchini
- 2 cloves garlic, minced
- 2 tbsp chopped fresh basil
- 2 tbsp grated Parmesan cheese
- 1 tbsp olive oil
- Salt and pepper to taste

Instructions:

1. Preheat oven to 400°F. Lightly grease a baking sheet.

2. Arrange the portobello mushroom caps, gill-side up, on the prepared baking sheet.

3. In a medium bowl, combine the chopped mushroom stems, cooked quinoa, bell peppers, onion, zucchini, garlic, basil, Parmesan, and olive oil. Season with salt and pepper.

4. Spoon the quinoa and vegetable mixture evenly into the portobello mushroom caps.

5. Bake for 18-22 minutes, until the mushrooms are tender and the filling is hot.

6. Serve the stuffed portobello mushrooms warm.

This dish is perfect for athletes as it provides complex carbs from the quinoa, fiber and nutrients from the vegetables, and a bit of protein from the Parmesan cheese. The portobello mushrooms add an earthy, meaty texture. It's a satisfying and nutrient-dense vegetarian meal.

You can customize the vegetables based on your preferences. Enjoy!

51. Baked cod with mango salsa and quinoa pilaf

Ingredients:
Mango Salsa:
- 1 ripe mango, diced
- 1/2 cup diced red onion
- 1/4 cup chopped fresh cilantro
- 1 jalapeño, seeded and minced (optional)
- 2 tbsp lime juice
- Salt and pepper to taste

Cod:
- 4 (6 oz) cod fillets
- 2 tbsp olive oil
- 1 tsp chili powder
- 1/2 tsp garlic powder
- Salt and pepper to taste

Quinoa Pilaf:
- 1 cup uncooked quinoa, rinsed
- 2 cups low-sodium chicken or vegetable broth
- 1 tbsp olive oil
- 1 onion, diced
- 2 cloves garlic, minced
- 1 tsp ground cumin
- 1/4 cup chopped fresh parsley

Instructions:
1. Make the mango salsa: In a bowl, combine the diced mango, red onion, cilantro, jalapeño (if using), and lime juice. Season with salt and pepper. Refrigerate until ready to serve.

2. Preheat oven to 400°F. Line a baking sheet with parchment paper.

3. Place the cod fillets on the prepared baking sheet. Drizzle with the 2 tbsp olive oil and sprinkle with the chili powder, garlic powder, salt, and pepper.

4. Bake the cod for 12-15 minutes, until it flakes easily with a fork.

5. Make the quinoa pilaf: In a medium saucepan, combine the quinoa and broth. Bring to a boil, then reduce heat and simmer for 15-20 minutes until quinoa is tender.

6. In a skillet, heat the 1 tbsp olive oil over medium heat. Sauté the onion and garlic for 3-4 minutes until fragrant.

7. Fluff the cooked quinoa with a fork and stir in the sautéed onion and garlic, cumin, and parsley. Serve the baked cod topped with the mango salsa, alongside the quinoa pilaf.

This meal is perfect for athletes as it provides lean protein from the cod, complex carbs from the quinoa, and healthy fats and nutrients from the mango salsa. It's a well-balanced and flavorful dish.

52. Turkey and vegetable lettuce wraps with hoisin sauce

Ingredients:
Filling:
- 1 lb ground turkey
- 1 tbsp sesame oil
- 2 cloves garlic, minced
- 1 tbsp grated fresh ginger
- 1 cup shredded carrots
- 1 cup shredded cabbage
- 1/2 cup diced water chestnuts
- 2 tbsp low-sodium soy sauce
- 1 tbsp rice vinegar
- Salt and pepper to taste

Hoisin Sauce:
- 1/4 cup hoisin sauce
- 1 tbsp rice vinegar
- 1 tsp sesame oil
- 1 tsp sriracha (optional)

To Serve:
- 12-16 large lettuce leaves (such as romaine or bibb)
- Chopped green onions for garnish

Instructions:

1. In a large skillet or wok, cook the ground turkey over medium-high heat, breaking it up with a wooden spoon, until browned, about 5-7 minutes. Drain any excess fat.

2. Add the sesame oil, garlic, and ginger to the pan. Cook for 1 minute until fragrant.

3. Stir in the shredded carrots, cabbage, water chestnuts, soy sauce, and rice vinegar. Season with salt and pepper.

4. In a small bowl, whisk together the ingredients for the hoisin sauce.

5. To serve, place a spoonful of the turkey and vegetable mixture into a lettuce leaf. Drizzle with the hoisin sauce and garnish with chopped green onions.

These turkey and vegetable lettuce wraps are perfect for athletes as they provide lean protein from the turkey, fiber and nutrients from the vegetables, and a flavorful sauce without too many calories. They're a light, refreshing, and nutritious meal.

53. Ratatouille with quinoa

Ingredients:
- 1 cup uncooked quinoa
- 2 cups vegetable broth
- 1 medium eggplant, diced
- 1 zucchini, diced
- 1 red bell pepper, diced
- 1 onion, diced
- 3 cloves garlic, minced
- 2 tomatoes, diced
- 2 tbsp olive oil
- 1 tsp dried thyme
- 1 tsp dried oregano
- Salt and pepper to taste
- Fresh basil for garnish (optional)

Instructions:

1. Cook the quinoa according to package instructions, using the vegetable broth instead of water. Set aside.

2. In a large skillet or Dutch oven, heat the olive oil over medium heat. Add the onion and sauté for 2-3 minutes until translucent.

3. Add the garlic, eggplant, zucchini, and bell pepper. Sauté for 5-7 minutes, stirring occasionally, until the vegetables start to soften.

4. Stir in the diced tomatoes, thyme, oregano, salt, and pepper. Simmer for 10-15 minutes, until the vegetables are tender.

5. Fluff the cooked quinoa with a fork and stir it into the ratatouille mixture.

6. Serve hot, garnished with fresh basil if desired.

This dish is packed with complex carbs from the quinoa, fiber and antioxidants from the vegetables, and healthy fats from the olive oil - making it an excellent choice for athletes looking for a nutrient-dense, plant-based meal.

54. Grilled lemon herb tilapia with roasted vegetables

Ingredients:
- 4 tilapia fillets (about 4-6 oz each)
- 2 tbsp olive oil
- 2 tbsp lemon juice
- 2 tsp dried oregano
- 1 tsp dried basil
- 1 tsp garlic powder
- Salt and pepper to taste

For the Roasted Vegetables:
- 1 lb Brussels sprouts, trimmed and halved
- 1 medium zucchini, sliced into half-moons
- 1 red bell pepper, diced
- 1 red onion, diced
- 2 tbsp olive oil
- 1 tsp dried thyme
- Salt and pepper to taste

Instructions:

1. Preheat grill or grill pan to medium-high heat.

2. In a shallow dish, combine the olive oil, lemon juice, oregano, basil, garlic powder, salt, and pepper. Add the tilapia fillets and turn to coat both sides.

3. For the roasted vegetables, toss the Brussels sprouts, zucchini, bell pepper, and onion with the olive oil, thyme, salt, and pepper on a large baking sheet.

4. Grill the tilapia for 3-4 minutes per side, until cooked through and flaky.

5. Roast the vegetables in the oven at 400°F for 20-25 minutes, stirring halfway, until tender and lightly browned.

6. Serve the grilled lemon herb tilapia with the roasted vegetables. Garnish with extra lemon wedges if desired.

This meal is high in lean protein from the tilapia, packed with fiber and nutrients from the roasted veggies, and provides a good balance of healthy fats, carbs, and protein - making it an excellent choice for active athletes.

55. Turkey and spinach stuffed acorn squash

Ingredients:
- 2 acorn squash, halved and seeded
- 1 lb ground turkey
- 1 onion, diced
- 3 cloves garlic, minced
- 5 oz fresh spinach, chopped
- 1/2 cup cooked quinoa
- 1 tsp dried oregano
- 1 tsp dried basil
- Salt and pepper to taste
- 1/4 cup shredded mozzarella cheese (optional)

Instructions:

1. Preheat oven to 400°F. Place the acorn squash halves cut-side down on a baking sheet. Roast for 30-40 minutes, until tender when pierced with a fork.

2. In a large skillet over medium heat, cook the ground turkey, breaking it up as it cooks, until no longer pink, about 5-7 minutes. Drain any excess fat.

3. Add the diced onion and minced garlic to the skillet. Sauté for 2-3 minutes until the onion is translucent.

4. Stir in the chopped spinach and cook for 2-3 minutes until wilted.

5. Remove the skillet from heat and stir in the cooked quinoa, oregano, basil, salt, and pepper.

6. Flip the roasted acorn squash halves over so they are cut-side up. Spoon the turkey and spinach mixture evenly into the squash cavities.

7. If desired, top the stuffed squash with the shredded mozzarella cheese.

8. Return the stuffed squash to the oven and bake for an additional 10-15 minutes, until the cheese is melted and bubbly.

9. Serve the turkey and spinach stuffed acorn squash warm.

This dish is packed with complex carbs from the acorn squash and quinoa, lean protein from the turkey, and nutrient-dense spinach - making it an excellent choice for athletes looking for a balanced, satisfying meal.

56. Chickpea and vegetable tagine with couscous

Ingredients:
- 1 cup dry couscous
- 1 1/4 cups vegetable broth
- 1 tbsp olive oil
- 1 onion, diced
- 3 cloves garlic, minced
- 1 tsp ground cumin
- 1 tsp ground coriander
- 1 tsp paprika
- 1/2 tsp ground cinnamon
- 1/4 tsp cayenne pepper (optional)
- 1 (15oz) can chickpeas, drained and rinsed
- 1 medium sweet potato, peeled and diced
- 1 zucchini, diced
- 1 red bell pepper, diced
- 1 (14.5oz) can diced tomatoes
- 1/4 cup chopped fresh cilantro
- Salt and pepper to taste

Instructions:

1. Bring the vegetable broth to a boil in a small saucepan. Stir in the couscous, cover, and remove from heat. Let sit for 5-10 minutes until liquid is absorbed.

2. In a large skillet or Dutch oven, heat the olive oil over medium heat. Add the onion and sauté for 2-3 minutes until translucent.

3. Stir in the garlic, cumin, coriander, paprika, cinnamon, and cayenne (if using). Cook for 1 minute until fragrant.

4. Add the chickpeas, sweet potato, zucchini, bell pepper, and diced tomatoes. Season with salt and pepper.

5. Bring the mixture to a simmer, then reduce heat and let cook for 15-20 minutes, stirring occasionally, until the vegetables are tender.

6. Fluff the cooked couscous with a fork. Serve the chickpea and vegetable tagine over the couscous, garnished with fresh cilantro.

This dish is high in complex carbs from the couscous and sweet potato, packed with fiber and nutrients from the vegetables, and provides plant-based protein from the chickpeas - making it an excellent choice for fueling active athletes.

57. Baked chicken thighs with ratatouille

Ingredients:
- 6 bone-in, skin-on chicken thighs
- 2 tbsp olive oil, divided
- 1 tsp dried thyme
- 1 tsp dried oregano
- Salt and pepper to taste

For the Ratatouille:
- 1 medium eggplant, diced
- 1 zucchini, diced
- 1 red bell pepper, diced

- 1 onion, diced
- 3 cloves garlic, minced
- 2 tomatoes, diced
- 2 tbsp olive oil
- 1 tsp dried thyme
- 1 tsp dried oregano
- Salt and pepper to taste
- Fresh basil for garnish (optional)

Instructions:

1. Preheat oven to 400°F.

2. Pat the chicken thighs dry and place them in a large baking dish. Drizzle with 1 tbsp olive oil and sprinkle with the thyme, oregano, salt, and pepper. Rub the seasoning all over the chicken.

3. Bake the chicken for 35-40 minutes, until the internal temperature reaches 165°F.

4. While the chicken is baking, make the ratatouille. In a large skillet, heat the remaining 1 tbsp olive oil over medium heat.

5. Add the diced eggplant, zucchini, bell pepper, and onion. Sauté for 5-7 minutes, stirring occasionally, until the vegetables start to soften.

6. Stir in the minced garlic, diced tomatoes, thyme, oregano, salt, and pepper. Simmer for 10-15 minutes, until the vegetables are tender.

7. Serve the baked chicken thighs over the ratatouille, garnished with fresh basil if desired.

This meal provides a balance of lean protein from the chicken, complex carbs and fiber from the ratatouille vegetables, and healthy fats from the olive oil - making it an excellent choice for active athletes.

58. Quinoa and black bean burgers with avocado

Ingredients:

- 1 cup cooked quinoa
- 1 (15oz) can black beans, drained and rinsed
- 1/2 cup rolled oats
- 1/4 cup finely chopped onion
- 2 cloves garlic, minced
- 1 tsp ground cumin
- 1 tsp chili powder
- 1/4 tsp cayenne pepper (optional)
- Salt and pepper to taste
- 1 avocado, sliced
- Whole wheat buns or lettuce wraps

Instructions:

1. In a large bowl, mash the black beans with a fork or potato masher until slightly chunky.

2. Add the cooked quinoa, rolled oats, onion, garlic, cumin, chili powder, cayenne (if using), salt, and pepper. Mix well until fully combined.

3. Divide the mixture into 4-6 equal portions and form them into patties, about 1/2 inch thick.

4. Heat a large skillet or grill pan over medium heat. Add a small amount of oil or cooking spray.

5. Cook the quinoa and black bean patties for 4-5 minutes per side, until lightly browned and heated through.

6. Serve the burgers on whole wheat buns or lettuce wraps, topped with sliced avocado.

These quinoa and black bean burgers are packed with plant-based protein, complex carbs, fiber, and healthy fats - making them an excellent choice for fueling active athletes. The avocado topping adds even more healthy fats and nutrients.

59. Tofu and vegetable pad thai

Ingredients:
- 8 oz rice noodles
- 2 tbsp vegetable oil
- 1 block (14 oz) extra-firm tofu, cubed
- 2 cloves garlic, minced
- 1 cup shredded carrots
- 1 cup bean sprouts
- 1 red bell pepper, thinly sliced
- 3 green onions, sliced
- 2 eggs, lightly beaten
- 3 tbsp fish sauce
- 2 tbsp lime juice
- 2 tbsp brown sugar
- 1 tsp chili-garlic sauce (or to taste)
- 1/4 cup chopped roasted peanuts
- Lime wedges for serving

Instructions:

1. Soak the rice noodles in hot water for 15-20 minutes until softened. Drain and set aside.

2. In a large skillet or wok, heat the vegetable oil over medium-high heat. Add the cubed tofu and cook for 3-4 minutes per side until lightly browned. Remove tofu from the pan and set aside.

3. In the same pan, add the minced garlic and sauté for 1 minute until fragrant.

4. Add the softened rice noodles, carrots, bean sprouts, bell pepper, and green onions. Stir-fry for 2-3 minutes.

5. Push the vegetables to the side of the pan and pour in the beaten eggs. Scramble the eggs for 1-2 minutes until cooked through.

6. Stir the eggs into the vegetable mixture. Add the fish sauce, lime juice, brown sugar, and chili-garlic sauce. Toss everything together until well combined.

7. Gently fold in the cooked tofu cubes. Serve the pad thai hot, garnished with chopped peanuts and lime wedges.

This tofu and vegetable pad thai is a nutritious, protein-packed meal that's perfect for fueling active athletes. The combination of rice noodles, tofu, and veggies provides complex carbs, lean protein, and essential vitamins and minerals.

60. Greek turkey and vegetable skewers with tzatziki sauce

Ingredients:
For the Skewers:
- 1 lb ground turkey
- 1 zucchini, cut into 1-inch pieces
- 1 red onion, cut into 1-inch pieces
- 1 red bell pepper, cut into 1-inch pieces
- 8 cherry tomatoes
- 2 tbsp olive oil
- 1 tsp dried oregano
- 1 tsp dried basil
- Salt and pepper to taste

For the Tzatziki Sauce:
- 1 cup plain Greek yogurt
- 1 cucumber, grated and squeezed dry
- 2 cloves garlic, minced
- 1 tbsp lemon juice
- 1 tsp dried dill
- Salt and pepper to taste

Instructions:
1. Preheat grill or grill pan to medium-high heat.

2. In a large bowl, combine the ground turkey, zucchini, onion, bell pepper, and cherry tomatoes. Drizzle with olive oil and sprinkle with oregano, basil, salt, and pepper. Toss to coat.

3. Thread the turkey and vegetable pieces onto skewers, alternating the ingredients.

4. Grill the skewers for 12-15 minutes, turning occasionally, until the turkey is cooked through and the vegetables are tender.

5. Meanwhile, make the tzatziki sauce. In a medium bowl, mix together the Greek yogurt, grated cucumber, garlic, lemon juice, dill, salt, and pepper.

6. Serve the grilled turkey and vegetable skewers with the tzatziki sauce on the side for dipping.

These Greek-inspired skewers provide a balance of lean protein from the turkey, complex carbs and fiber from the vegetables, and healthy fats from the olive oil and yogurt-based tzatziki sauce - making it an excellent meal for active athletes.

61. Lentil and vegetable stuffed peppers with tomato sauce

Ingredients:
For the Stuffed Peppers:
- 6 bell peppers, halved and seeded
- 1 cup cooked lentils
- 1 cup cooked quinoa
- 1 cup diced zucchini
- 1/2 cup diced onion
- 2 cloves garlic, minced
- 1 tsp dried oregano
- 1 tsp dried basil
- Salt and pepper to taste

For the Tomato Sauce:
- 1 (28oz) can crushed tomatoes
- 2 cloves garlic, minced
- 1 tsp dried oregano
- 1 tsp dried basil
- Salt and pepper to taste

Instructions:
1. Preheat oven to 375°F.

2. In a large bowl, combine the cooked lentils, quinoa, zucchini, onion, garlic, oregano, basil, salt, and pepper. Mix well.

3. Stuff the lentil and vegetable mixture into the hollowed-out bell pepper halves, packing it in tightly.

4. Arrange the stuffed pepper halves in a baking dish.

5. In a medium saucepan, combine the crushed tomatoes, garlic, oregano, basil, salt, and pepper. Bring to a simmer.

6. Pour the tomato sauce over and around the stuffed peppers.

7. Cover the baking dish with foil and bake for 30-35 minutes, until the peppers are tender.

8. Remove the foil and bake for an additional 10 minutes to allow the tops to brown slightly.

9. Serve the lentil and vegetable stuffed peppers warm, with the tomato sauce spooned over the top.

This dish is packed with plant-based protein from the lentils and quinoa, fiber and nutrients from the vegetables, and antioxidants from the tomato sauce - making it an excellent choice for fueling active athletes.

62. Baked salmon with mango avocado salsa and quinoa

Ingredients:
- 4 salmon fillets (about 6 oz each)
- 1 cup uncooked quinoa
- 1 mango, diced
- 1 avocado, diced
- 1/2 red onion, finely chopped
- 1 jalapeño, seeded and finely chopped
- 1/4 cup chopped cilantro
- Juice of 1 lime
- Salt and pepper to taste

Instructions:

1. Preheat oven to 400°F. Line a baking sheet with parchment paper.

2. Place the salmon fillets on the prepared baking sheet and season with salt and pepper. Bake for 12-15 minutes, until salmon is cooked through.

3. Meanwhile, cook the quinoa according to package instructions. Fluff with a fork and set aside.

4. In a medium bowl, combine the diced mango, avocado, red onion, jalapeño, cilantro, and lime juice. Season with salt and pepper.

5. To serve, place a portion of quinoa on a plate. Top with a baked salmon fillet and spoon the mango avocado salsa over the top.

This dish is packed with lean protein from the salmon, complex carbs from the quinoa, and healthy fats and antioxidants from the mango and avocado. It's a nutritious and delicious meal for active individuals.

63. Chicken and vegetable lettuce cups with peanut sauce

Ingredients:

- 1 lb boneless, skinless chicken breasts, diced
- 2 cups mixed vegetables (such as shredded carrots, sliced bell peppers, shredded cabbage)
- 8-10 large lettuce leaves (such as romaine or bibb)
- 1/4 cup creamy peanut butter
- 2 tbsp low-sodium soy sauce
- 2 tbsp rice vinegar
- 1 tbsp honey
- 1 tsp sesame oil
- 1 garlic clove, minced
- 1-2 tbsp water to thin the sauce

Instructions:

1. In a large skillet or wok, cook the diced chicken over medium-high heat until no longer pink, about 6-8 minutes. Transfer to a bowl.

2. In the same skillet, sauté the mixed vegetables for 3-4 minutes until tender-crisp.

3. In a small bowl, whisk together the peanut butter, soy sauce, rice vinegar, honey, sesame oil, and garlic. Add water as needed to thin the sauce to a pourable consistency.

4. To assemble, place a spoonful of the chicken and vegetable mixture into each lettuce leaf. Drizzle the peanut sauce over the top.

5. Serve the lettuce cups immediately, allowing guests to customize their own.

This dish is a great source of lean protein, fiber, and healthy fats. The peanut sauce adds a delicious flavor boost. It's a nutritious and portable meal option for active individuals.

64. Quinoa and black bean stuffed sweet potatoes

Ingredients:
- 4 medium sweet potatoes
- 1 cup cooked quinoa
- 1 (15 oz) can black beans, drained and rinsed
- 1/2 cup diced red onion
- 1 jalapeño, seeded and diced (optional)
- 1 tsp ground cumin
- 1 tsp chili powder
- 1/4 cup chopped cilantro
- Salt and pepper to taste
- Toppings (optional): avocado, salsa, Greek yogurt, etc.

Instructions:

1. Preheat oven to 400°F. Pierce the sweet potatoes several times with a fork and place on a baking sheet. Bake for 45-60 minutes, until very soft when squeezed.

2. In a medium bowl, combine the cooked quinoa, black beans, red onion, jalapeño (if using), cumin, chili powder, and cilantro. Season with salt and pepper.

3. Once the sweet potatoes are cooked, let them cool slightly. Slice each potato in half lengthwise and scoop out the flesh, leaving about 1/4 inch of the potato skin intact.

4. Mash the sweet potato flesh and fold it into the quinoa and black bean mixture until well combined.

5. Spoon the quinoa and black bean mixture back into the sweet potato skins.

6. Return the stuffed sweet potatoes to the oven and bake for an additional 10-15 minutes, until heated through.

7. Serve the stuffed sweet potatoes warm, with desired toppings.

This dish is a nutritious and satisfying meal for athletes, providing complex carbs, protein, fiber, and essential vitamins and minerals.

65. Grilled shrimp and vegetable kabobs with quinoa

Ingredients:
- 1 lb large shrimp, peeled and deveined
- 1 zucchini, cut into 1-inch pieces
- 1 red bell pepper, cut into 1-inch pieces
- 1 red onion, cut into 1-inch pieces
- 8 oz mushrooms, halved
- 1 cup uncooked quinoa
- 2 tbsp olive oil
- 2 tbsp lemon juice
- 1 tsp dried oregano
- 1 tsp garlic powder
- Salt and pepper to taste

Instructions:

1. Preheat grill to medium-high heat.

2. In a large bowl, combine the shrimp, zucchini, bell pepper, onion, and mushrooms. Drizzle with olive oil, lemon juice, oregano, garlic powder, salt, and pepper. Toss to coat.

3. Thread the shrimp and vegetables onto skewers, alternating the ingredients.

4. Grill the kabobs for 12-15 minutes, turning occasionally, until the shrimp are opaque and the vegetables are tender.

5. Meanwhile, cook the quinoa according to package instructions. Fluff with a fork.

6. Serve the grilled shrimp and vegetable kabobs over the cooked quinoa.

This dish is packed with lean protein from the shrimp, complex carbs from the quinoa, and a variety of nutrient-dense vegetables. It's a well-balanced and flavorful meal for active individuals.

66. Turkey and vegetable stuffed zucchini boats

Ingredients:
- 4 medium zucchini, halved lengthwise
- 1 lb ground turkey
- 1 cup diced onion
- 1 cup diced bell pepper
- 2 cloves garlic, minced
- 1 tsp dried oregano
- 1 tsp dried basil
- 1/2 tsp red pepper flakes (optional)
- Salt and pepper to taste
- 1 cup shredded mozzarella cheese

Instructions:

1. Preheat oven to 400°F. Scoop out the flesh from the zucchini halves, leaving about 1/4 inch of the zucchini shell. Finely chop the scooped out zucchini flesh.

2. In a large skillet over medium heat, cook the ground turkey, breaking it up as it cooks, until no longer pink, about 5-7 minutes. Drain any excess fat.

3. Add the chopped zucchini flesh, onion, bell pepper, garlic, oregano, basil, red pepper flakes (if using), salt, and pepper to the skillet. Cook for 5-7 minutes, until the vegetables are tender.

4. Arrange the zucchini boats in a baking dish. Spoon the turkey and vegetable mixture evenly into the zucchini boats.

5. Top each stuffed zucchini boat with shredded mozzarella cheese.

6. Bake for 20-25 minutes, until the zucchini is tender and the cheese is melted and bubbly.

7. Serve the stuffed zucchini boats warm.

This dish is a great source of lean protein, fiber, and essential vitamins and minerals. The zucchini boats provide a low-carb, nutrient-dense vessel for the flavorful turkey and vegetable filling, making it a perfect meal for athletes.

67. Tofu and vegetable stir-fry with brown rice

Ingredients:
- 1 cup uncooked brown rice
- 1 block (14 oz) extra-firm tofu, cubed
- 2 tbsp sesame oil
- 2 cups mixed vegetables (such as broccoli, carrots, snow peas, bell peppers)
- 2 cloves garlic, minced
- 1 tbsp grated fresh ginger
- 2 tbsp low-sodium soy sauce
- 1 tbsp rice vinegar
- 1 tsp honey
- 1/4 tsp red pepper flakes (optional)
- Salt and pepper to taste
- Chopped green onions and sesame seeds for garnish (optional)

Instructions:

1. Cook the brown rice according to package instructions. Set aside.

2. In a large skillet or wok, heat the sesame oil over medium-high heat. Add the cubed tofu and cook for 5-7 minutes, turning occasionally, until lightly browned on all sides. Transfer the tofu to a plate.

3. In the same skillet, add the mixed vegetables, garlic, and ginger. Stir-fry for 5-7 minutes, until the vegetables are tender-crisp.

4. Return the tofu to the skillet. Add the soy sauce, rice vinegar, honey, and red pepper flakes (if using). Toss to coat everything evenly.

5. Serve the tofu and vegetable stir-fry over the cooked brown rice. Garnish with chopped green onions and sesame seeds, if desired.

This dish is a great source of plant-based protein from the tofu, complex carbs from the brown rice, and a variety of nutrient-dense vegetables. It's a well-balanced and flavorful meal for active individuals.

68. Greek-style baked chicken with roasted vegetables and couscous

Ingredients:

- 4 boneless, skinless chicken breasts
- 2 tbsp olive oil
- 2 tsp dried oregano
- 1 tsp garlic powder
- 1 tsp lemon zest
- Salt and pepper to taste
- 2 cups mixed vegetables (such as diced zucchini, bell peppers, onions, and cherry tomatoes)
- 1 cup uncooked couscous
- 1 cup low-sodium chicken broth
- 2 tbsp crumbled feta cheese
- 2 tbsp chopped fresh parsley

Instructions:

1. Preheat oven to 400°F. Line a baking sheet with parchment paper.

2. In a small bowl, combine the olive oil, oregano, garlic powder, lemon zest, salt, and pepper. Rub the mixture all over the chicken breasts.

3. Place the chicken on the prepared baking sheet. Arrange the mixed vegetables around the chicken.

4. Bake for 25-30 minutes, or until the chicken is cooked through and the vegetables are tender.

5. Meanwhile, prepare the couscous according to package instructions, using the chicken broth instead of water.

6. Fluff the cooked couscous with a fork and stir in the crumbled feta and chopped parsley.

7. Serve the baked chicken and roasted vegetables over the Greek-style couscous.

This dish is a well-balanced meal for athletes, providing lean protein from the chicken, complex carbs from the couscous, and a variety of nutrient-dense vegetables. The Greek-inspired flavors make it a delicious and satisfying option.

69. Lentil and vegetable curry with quinoa

Ingredients:
- 1 cup uncooked quinoa
- 1 tbsp olive oil
- 1 onion, diced
- 3 cloves garlic, minced
- 1 tbsp grated fresh ginger
- 2 tsp curry powder
- 1 tsp ground cumin
- 1/2 tsp ground turmeric
- 1/4 tsp cayenne pepper (optional)
- 1 cup red lentils, rinsed
- 1 (14 oz) can diced tomatoes
- 2 cups low-sodium vegetable broth
- 2 cups mixed vegetables (such as cauliflower, spinach, peas)
- 1 (13.5 oz) can full-fat coconut milk
- Salt and pepper to taste
- Chopped cilantro for garnish

Instructions:

1. Cook the quinoa according to package instructions. Fluff with a fork and set aside.

2. In a large pot or Dutch oven, heat the olive oil over medium heat. Add the onion and sauté for 3-4 minutes until translucent.

3. Add the garlic, ginger, curry powder, cumin, turmeric, and cayenne (if using). Cook for 1 minute, stirring constantly, until fragrant.

4. Stir in the lentils, diced tomatoes, and vegetable broth. Bring to a boil, then reduce heat and simmer for 15-20 minutes, until the lentils are tender.

5. Add the mixed vegetables and coconut milk. Simmer for an additional 5-7 minutes, until the vegetables are tender.

6. Season the curry with salt and pepper to taste. Serve the lentil and vegetable curry over the cooked quinoa. Garnish with chopped cilantro.

This dish is packed with plant-based protein from the lentils, complex carbs from the quinoa, and a variety of nutrient-dense vegetables. It's a flavorful and satisfying meal for active individuals.

70. Black bean and corn stuffed bell peppers with avocado

Ingredients:
- 4 bell peppers, halved lengthwise and seeds removed
- 1 (15 oz) can black beans, drained and rinsed
- 1 cup frozen corn, thawed
- 1/2 cup cooked quinoa
- 1/2 cup diced onion
- 2 cloves garlic, minced
- 1 tsp chili powder
- 1/2 tsp cumin
- Salt and pepper to taste
- 1 avocado, diced
- Chopped cilantro for garnish

Instructions:

1. Preheat oven to 375°F. Place the bell pepper halves in a baking dish and set aside.

2. In a medium bowl, combine the black beans, corn, quinoa, onion, garlic, chili powder, cumin, salt, and pepper. Stir to mix well.

3. Spoon the black bean and corn mixture evenly into the bell pepper halves.

4. Cover the baking dish with foil and bake for 25-30 minutes, until the peppers are tender.

5. Remove the foil and bake for an additional 5 minutes to lightly brown the tops.

6. Top the stuffed bell peppers with the diced avocado and chopped cilantro.

7. Serve the stuffed bell peppers warm.

This dish is a nutritious and satisfying meal for athletes, providing a balance of complex carbs, protein, fiber, and healthy fats. The bell peppers provide a nutrient-dense vessel for the flavorful black bean and corn filling.

71. Teriyaki tofu and vegetable stir-fry with soba noodles

Ingredients:
- 8 oz soba noodles
- 1 block (14 oz) extra-firm tofu, cubed
- 2 tbsp sesame oil, divided
- 2 cups mixed vegetables (such as broccoli, carrots, snow peas, bell peppers)
- 2 cloves garlic, minced
- 1 tbsp grated fresh ginger
- 1/4 cup low-sodium teriyaki sauce
- 2 tbsp low-sodium soy sauce
- 1 tsp honey
- Salt and pepper to taste
- Chopped green onions and sesame seeds for garnish (optional)

Instructions:

1. Cook the soba noodles according to package instructions. Drain and set aside.

2. In a large skillet or wok, heat 1 tbsp of the sesame oil over medium-high heat. Add the cubed tofu and cook for 5-7 minutes, turning occasionally, until lightly browned on all sides. Transfer the tofu to a plate.

3. In the same skillet, heat the remaining 1 tbsp of sesame oil. Add the mixed vegetables, garlic, and ginger. Stir-fry for 5-7 minutes, until the vegetables are tender-crisp.

4. Return the tofu to the skillet. Add the teriyaki sauce, soy sauce, and honey. Toss to coat everything evenly and heat through.

5. Add the cooked soba noodles to the skillet and toss to combine.

6. Serve the teriyaki tofu and vegetable stir-fry with soba noodles, garnished with chopped green onions and sesame seeds, if desired.

This dish is a great source of plant-based protein from the tofu, complex carbs from the soba noodles, and a variety of nutrient-dense vegetables. It's a well-balanced and flavorful meal for active individuals.

72. Mediterranean–style baked cod with quinoa salad

Ingredients:
For the Baked Cod:
- 4 (6 oz) cod fillets
- 2 tbsp olive oil
- 2 cloves garlic, minced
- 1 tsp dried oregano
- 1 tsp paprika
- Zest of 1 lemon
- Salt and pepper to taste

For the Quinoa Salad:
- 1 cup uncooked quinoa, cooked according to package instructions
- 1 cup diced cucumber
- 1 cup cherry tomatoes, halved
- 1/2 cup diced red onion
- 1/4 cup crumbled feta cheese
- 2 tbsp chopped fresh parsley
- 2 tbsp lemon juice
- 1 tbsp olive oil
- Salt and pepper to taste

Instructions:
1. Preheat oven to 400°F. Line a baking sheet with parchment paper.

2. In a small bowl, combine the olive oil, garlic, oregano, paprika, lemon zest, salt, and pepper. Rub the mixture over the cod fillets.

3. Place the cod fillets on the prepared baking sheet. Bake for 12-15 minutes, until the fish flakes easily with a fork.

4. While the cod is baking, prepare the quinoa salad. In a large bowl, combine the cooked quinoa, cucumber, tomatoes, red onion, feta, and parsley.

5. Drizzle the lemon juice and olive oil over the quinoa salad. Season with salt and pepper, and toss to coat. Serve the baked cod fillets over the Mediterranean-style quinoa salad.

This dish is a great source of lean protein from the cod, complex carbs from the quinoa, and healthy fats and antioxidants from the vegetables and olive oil. It's a well-balanced and flavorful meal for active individuals.

73. Turkey and vegetable kebabs with quinoa

Ingredients:
- 1 lb ground turkey
- 1 zucchini, cut into 1-inch pieces
- 1 red bell pepper, cut into 1-inch pieces
- 1 red onion, cut into 1-inch pieces
- 8 oz mushrooms, halved
- 1 cup uncooked quinoa
- 2 tbsp olive oil
- 2 tbsp lemon juice
- 1 tsp dried oregano
- 1 tsp garlic powder
- Salt and pepper to taste

Instructions:

1. Preheat grill to medium-high heat.

2. In a large bowl, combine the ground turkey, zucchini, bell pepper, onion, and mushrooms. Drizzle with olive oil, lemon juice, oregano, garlic powder, salt, and pepper. Mix well until everything is evenly coated.

3. Thread the turkey and vegetable pieces onto skewers, alternating the ingredients.

4. Grill the kebabs for 12-15 minutes, turning occasionally, until the turkey is cooked through and the vegetables are tender.

5. Meanwhile, cook the quinoa according to package instructions. Fluff with a fork.

6. Serve the grilled turkey and vegetable kebabs over the cooked quinoa.

This dish is a great source of lean protein from the turkey, complex carbs from the quinoa, and a variety of nutrient-dense vegetables. It's a well-balanced and flavorful meal for active individuals.

74. Chickpea and vegetable tikka masala with brown rice

Ingredients:

- 1 cup uncooked brown rice
- 1 (15 oz) can chickpeas, drained and rinsed
- 2 cups mixed vegetables (such as cauliflower, bell peppers, onions)
- 2 tbsp olive oil
- 2 cloves garlic, minced
- 1 tbsp grated fresh ginger
- 2 tsp garam masala
- 1 tsp ground cumin
- 1 tsp paprika
- 1/4 tsp cayenne pepper (optional)
- 1 (14 oz) can diced tomatoes
- 1 cup low-sodium vegetable broth
- 1/2 cup full-fat coconut milk
- Salt and pepper to taste
- Chopped cilantro for garnish

Instructions:

1. Cook the brown rice according to package instructions. Set aside.

2. In a large skillet or wok, heat the olive oil over medium heat. Add the chickpeas and mixed vegetables. Sauté for 5-7 minutes, until the vegetables are tender-crisp.

3. Add the garlic, ginger, garam masala, cumin, paprika, and cayenne (if using). Cook for 1-2 minutes, stirring constantly, until fragrant.

4. Pour in the diced tomatoes and vegetable broth. Bring the mixture to a simmer and let it cook for 10-15 minutes, until the sauce has thickened slightly.

5. Stir in the coconut milk and season with salt and pepper to taste.

6. Serve the chickpea and vegetable tikka masala over the cooked brown rice, garnished with chopped cilantro.

This dish is a great source of plant-based protein from the chickpeas, complex carbs from the brown rice, and a variety of nutrient-dense vegetables. The creamy, flavorful tikka masala sauce makes it a delicious and satisfying meal for athletes.

75. Greek-style grilled shrimp with orzo and roasted vegetables

Ingredients:
- 1 lb large shrimp, peeled and deveined
- 2 tbsp olive oil, divided
- 2 tsp dried oregano
- 1 tsp lemon zest
- Salt and pepper to taste
- 1 cup uncooked orzo pasta
- 2 cups mixed vegetables (such as zucchini, bell peppers, red onion), cut into 1-inch pieces
- 1/4 cup crumbled feta cheese
- 2 tbsp chopped fresh parsley
- 1 tbsp lemon juice

Instructions:

1. Preheat grill to medium-high heat.

2. In a large bowl, combine the shrimp, 1 tbsp of the olive oil, oregano, lemon zest, salt, and pepper. Toss to coat the shrimp evenly.

3. Thread the seasoned shrimp onto skewers.

4. In a separate bowl, toss the mixed vegetables with the remaining 1 tbsp of olive oil, salt, and pepper.

5. Grill the shrimp skewers and the vegetable mixture for 8-10 minutes, turning occasionally, until the shrimp are opaque and the vegetables are tender.

6. Meanwhile, cook the orzo according to package instructions. Drain and set aside.

7. In a large bowl, combine the cooked orzo, grilled vegetables, feta cheese, parsley, and lemon juice. Toss to mix well.

8. Serve the grilled shrimp skewers over the Greek-style orzo and vegetable salad.

This dish is a great source of lean protein from the shrimp, complex carbs from the orzo, and a variety of nutrient-dense vegetables. The Greek-inspired flavors make it a delicious and satisfying meal for active individuals.

76. Lentil and vegetable shepherd's pie with mashed sweet potatoes

Ingredients:
For the Filling:
- 1 cup dry brown or green lentils, rinsed
- 2 cups low-sodium vegetable broth
- 1 tbsp olive oil
- 1 onion, diced
- 2 carrots, diced
- 2 celery stalks, diced
- 3 cloves garlic, minced
- 1 tsp dried thyme
- 1 tsp dried rosemary
- 1 (14 oz) can diced tomatoes
- Salt and pepper to taste

For the Topping:
- 3 medium sweet potatoes, peeled and cubed
- 2 tbsp unsweetened almond milk
- 1 tbsp olive oil
- Salt and pepper to taste

Instructions:
1. Preheat oven to 375°F.

2. In a medium saucepan, combine the lentils and vegetable broth. Bring to a boil, then reduce heat and simmer for 20-25 minutes, until the lentils are tender. Drain any excess liquid and set aside.

3. In a large skillet, heat the olive oil over medium heat. Add the onion, carrots, celery, and garlic. Sauté for 5-7 minutes, until the vegetables are tender.

4. Stir in the cooked lentils, thyme, rosemary, and diced tomatoes. Season with salt and pepper to taste.

5. Transfer the lentil and vegetable mixture to a 9x13 inch baking dish.

6. In a medium saucepan, cover the sweet potato cubes with water and bring to a boil. Reduce heat and simmer for 15-20 minutes, until the sweet potatoes are very soft. Drain and return to the saucepan.

7. Mash the sweet potatoes with the almond milk and olive oil. Season with salt and pepper. Spread the mashed sweet potatoes evenly over the lentil and vegetable filling.

8. Bake for 25-30 minutes, until the topping is lightly browned. Let the shepherd's pie cool for 5-10 minutes before serving.

This dish is a nutritious and satisfying meal for athletes, providing plant-based protein, complex carbs, fiber, and essential vitamins and minerals.

77. Quinoa and black bean salad with avocado and lime dressing

Ingredients:
- 1 cup uncooked quinoa, cooked according to package instructions
- 1 (15 oz) can black beans, drained and rinsed
- 1 cup diced cucumber
- 1 cup cherry tomatoes, halved
- 1/2 cup diced red onion
- 1/4 cup chopped fresh cilantro
- 1 avocado, diced

For the Dressing:
- 1 avocado, mashed
- 2 tbsp lime juice
- 1 tbsp olive oil
- 1 tsp honey
- 1 clove garlic, minced
- Salt and pepper to taste

Instructions:

1. In a large bowl, combine the cooked quinoa, black beans, cucumber, tomatoes, red onion, and cilantro.

2. In a small bowl, mash the avocado for the dressing. Whisk in the lime juice, olive oil, honey, and garlic. Season with salt and pepper.

3. Pour the avocado lime dressing over the quinoa and black bean salad. Toss gently to coat.

4. Gently fold in the diced avocado.

5. Serve the quinoa and black bean salad chilled or at room temperature.

This salad is a nutritious and flavorful option for athletes, providing a balance of complex carbs, protein, fiber, and healthy fats. The avocado lime dressing adds a creamy, tangy flavor that complements the other ingredients.

78. Tofu and vegetable lettuce wraps with hoisin sauce

Ingredients:

- 1 block (14 oz) extra-firm tofu, diced
- 2 tbsp sesame oil, divided
- 2 cups mixed vegetables (such as shredded carrots, sliced bell peppers, shredded cabbage)
- 2 cloves garlic, minced
- 1 tbsp grated fresh ginger
- 2 tbsp hoisin sauce
- 1 tbsp low-sodium soy sauce
- 1 tsp rice vinegar
- 12-16 large lettuce leaves (such as romaine or bibb)
- Chopped green onions and toasted sesame seeds for garnish (optional)

Instructions:

1. In a large skillet or wok, heat 1 tbsp of the sesame oil over medium-high heat. Add the diced tofu and cook for 5-7 minutes, turning occasionally, until lightly browned on all sides. Transfer the tofu to a plate.

2. In the same skillet, heat the remaining 1 tbsp of sesame oil. Add the mixed vegetables, garlic, and ginger. Sauté for 3-4 minutes, until the vegetables are tender-crisp.

3. Return the cooked tofu to the skillet. Add the hoisin sauce, soy sauce, and rice vinegar. Toss to coat everything evenly and heat through.

4. To serve, place a spoonful of the tofu and vegetable mixture into each lettuce leaf. Garnish with chopped green onions and toasted sesame seeds, if desired.

These tofu and vegetable lettuce wraps are a great source of plant-based protein, fiber, and essential vitamins and minerals. The hoisin sauce adds a delicious savory-sweet flavor. This is a nutritious and portable meal option for active individuals.

79. Moroccan chickpea stew with couscous

Ingredients:
* 1 cup uncooked couscous
* 1 tbsp olive oil
* 1 onion, diced
* 3 cloves garlic, minced
* 1 tbsp grated fresh ginger
* 2 tsp ground cumin
* 1 tsp ground coriander
* 1 tsp paprika
* 1/2 tsp ground cinnamon
* 1/4 tsp cayenne pepper (optional)
* 1 (15 oz) can chickpeas, drained and rinsed
* 1 (14 oz) can diced tomatoes
* 2 cups low-sodium vegetable broth
* 1 cup diced sweet potato
* 1 cup frozen peas
* Salt and pepper to taste
* Chopped cilantro for garnish

Instructions:

1. Prepare the couscous according to package instructions. Fluff with a fork and set aside.

2. In a large pot or Dutch oven, heat the olive oil over medium heat. Add the onion and sauté for 3-4 minutes until translucent.

3. Add the garlic, ginger, cumin, coriander, paprika, cinnamon, and cayenne (if using). Cook for 1 minute, stirring constantly, until fragrant.

4. Stir in the chickpeas, diced tomatoes, vegetable broth, and sweet potato. Bring the mixture to a boil, then reduce heat and simmer for 15-20 minutes, until the sweet potato is tender.

5. Add the frozen peas and cook for an additional 5 minutes. Season the stew with salt and pepper to taste. Serve the Moroccan chickpea stew over the cooked couscous, garnished with chopped cilantro.

This dish is a nutritious and flavorful option for athletes, providing plant-based protein, complex carbs, fiber, and a variety of essential vitamins and minerals. The Moroccan-inspired spices add depth of flavor.

80. Baked salmon with lemon dill sauce and roasted vegetables

Ingredients:

For the Salmon:
- 4 (6 oz) salmon fillets
- 1 tbsp olive oil
- 1 tsp lemon zest
- Salt and pepper to taste

For the Lemon Dill Sauce:
- 1/2 cup plain Greek yogurt
- 2 tbsp lemon juice
- 1 tbsp chopped fresh dill
- 1 clove garlic, minced
- Salt and pepper to taste

For the Roasted Vegetables:
- 2 cups mixed vegetables (such as broccoli, carrots, Brussels sprouts, red onion), cut into 1-inch pieces
- 2 tbsp olive oil
- Salt and pepper to taste

Instructions:

1. Preheat oven to 400°F. Line a baking sheet with parchment paper.

2. Place the salmon fillets on the prepared baking sheet. Drizzle with olive oil and sprinkle with lemon zest, salt, and pepper.

3. In a small bowl, whisk together the ingredients for the lemon dill sauce. Set aside.

4. In a separate bowl, toss the mixed vegetables with olive oil, salt, and pepper.

5. Arrange the seasoned vegetables on the baking sheet around the salmon fillets.

6. Bake for 15-20 minutes, until the salmon is cooked through and the vegetables are tender.

7. Serve the baked salmon with the lemon dill sauce drizzled over the top. Enjoy the roasted vegetables on the side.

This dish is a nutritious and well-balanced meal for athletes, providing lean protein from the salmon, complex carbs and fiber from the roasted vegetables, and healthy fats from the olive oil and salmon. The lemon dill sauce adds a refreshing flavor.

81. Turkey and vegetable stir-fry with brown rice

Ingredients:
- 1 cup uncooked brown rice
- 1 lb ground turkey
- 2 tbsp sesame oil, divided
- 2 cups mixed vegetables (such as broccoli, bell peppers, snow peas, mushrooms)
- 2 cloves garlic, minced
- 1 tbsp grated fresh ginger
- 2 tbsp low-sodium soy sauce
- 1 tbsp rice vinegar
- 1 tsp honey
- Salt and pepper to taste
- Chopped green onions and toasted sesame seeds for garnish (optional)

Instructions:

1. Cook the brown rice according to package instructions. Set aside.

2. In a large skillet or wok, heat 1 tbsp of the sesame oil over medium-high heat. Add the ground turkey and cook, breaking it up as it cooks, until no longer pink, about 5-7 minutes. Transfer the cooked turkey to a plate.

3. In the same skillet, heat the remaining 1 tbsp of sesame oil. Add the mixed vegetables, garlic, and ginger. Stir-fry for 5-7 minutes, until the vegetables are tender-crisp.

4. Return the cooked turkey to the skillet. Add the soy sauce, rice vinegar, and honey. Toss to coat everything evenly and heat through.

5. Serve the turkey and vegetable stir-fry over the cooked brown rice. Garnish with chopped green onions and toasted sesame seeds, if desired.

This dish is a great source of lean protein from the turkey, complex carbs from the brown rice, and a variety of nutrient-dense vegetables. It's a well-balanced and flavorful meal for active individuals.

82. Greek turkey burgers
with tzatziki sauce and sweet potato fries

Ingredients:
For the Turkey Burgers:
- 1 lb ground turkey
- 2 tbsp crumbled feta cheese
- 2 tbsp chopped fresh parsley
- 1 tsp dried oregano
- 1 clove garlic, minced
- Salt and pepper to taste
- 4 whole wheat buns

For the Tzatziki Sauce:
- 1 cup plain Greek yogurt
- 1/2 cucumber, grated and squeezed dry
- 1 clove garlic, minced
- 1 tbsp lemon juice
- 1 tsp chopped fresh dill
- Salt and pepper to taste

For the Sweet Potato Fries:
- 2 medium sweet potatoes, cut into 1/2-inch thick fries
- 1 tbsp olive oil
- Salt and pepper to taste

Instructions:
1. Preheat oven to 400°F. Line a baking sheet with parchment paper.

2. In a large bowl, combine the ground turkey, feta, parsley, oregano, garlic, salt, and pepper. Mix well and form into 4 patties.

3. In a small bowl, mix together all the ingredients for the tzatziki sauce. Refrigerate until ready to serve.

4. Toss the sweet potato fries with the olive oil, salt, and pepper. Spread in a single layer on the prepared baking sheet.

5. Bake the sweet potato fries for 20-25 minutes, flipping halfway, until crispy.

6. Meanwhile, cook the turkey burgers in a skillet or on a grill over medium heat for 5-7 minutes per side, until cooked through.

7. Serve the Greek turkey burgers on the whole wheat buns, topped with the tzatziki sauce. Enjoy the sweet potato fries on the side.

This meal provides a balance of lean protein, complex carbs, and healthy fats to fuel active individuals. The Greek-inspired flavors make it a delicious and satisfying option.

83. Lentil and vegetable curry with quinoa

Ingredients:
- 1 cup uncooked quinoa
- 1 tbsp olive oil
- 1 onion, diced
- 3 cloves garlic, minced
- 1 tbsp grated fresh ginger
- 2 tsp curry powder
- 1 tsp ground cumin
- 1/2 tsp ground turmeric
- 1/4 tsp cayenne pepper (optional)
- 1 cup red lentils, rinsed
- 1 (14 oz) can diced tomatoes
- 2 cups low-sodium vegetable broth
- 2 cups mixed vegetables (such as cauliflower, spinach, peas)
- 1 (13.5 oz) can full-fat coconut milk
- Salt and pepper to taste
- Chopped cilantro for garnish

Instructions:

1. Cook the quinoa according to package instructions. Fluff with a fork and set aside.

2. In a large pot or Dutch oven, heat the olive oil over medium heat. Add the onion and sauté for 3-4 minutes until translucent.

3. Add the garlic, ginger, curry powder, cumin, turmeric, and cayenne (if using). Cook for 1 minute, stirring constantly, until fragrant.

4. Stir in the lentils, diced tomatoes, and vegetable broth. Bring to a boil, then reduce heat and simmer for 15-20 minutes, until the lentils are tender.

5. Add the mixed vegetables and coconut milk. Simmer for an additional 5-7 minutes, until the vegetables are tender.

6. Season the curry with salt and pepper to taste. Serve the lentil and vegetable curry over the cooked quinoa. Garnish with chopped cilantro.

This dish is packed with plant-based protein from the lentils, complex carbs from the quinoa, and a variety of nutrient-dense vegetables. It's a flavorful and satisfying meal for active individuals.

84. Tofu and vegetable pad thai

Ingredients:

- 8 oz rice noodles
- 1 block (14 oz) extra-firm tofu, cubed
- 2 tbsp sesame oil, divided
- 2 cups mixed vegetables (such as shredded carrots, bean sprouts, chopped cabbage, sliced bell peppers)
- 2 cloves garlic, minced
- 2 tbsp low-sodium soy sauce
- 2 tbsp rice vinegar
- 2 tbsp creamy peanut butter
- 1 tbsp honey
- 1 tsp chili garlic sauce (or sriracha)
- 2 eggs, lightly beaten
- 2 tbsp chopped roasted peanuts
- 2 tbsp chopped fresh cilantro

Instructions:

1. Prepare the rice noodles according to package instructions. Drain and set aside.

2. In a large skillet or wok, heat 1 tbsp of the sesame oil over medium-high heat. Add the cubed tofu and cook for 5-7 minutes, turning occasionally, until lightly browned on all sides. Transfer the tofu to a plate.

3. In the same skillet, heat the remaining 1 tbsp of sesame oil. Add the mixed vegetables and garlic. Stir-fry for 3-4 minutes, until the vegetables are tender-crisp.

4. In a small bowl, whisk together the soy sauce, rice vinegar, peanut butter, honey, and chili garlic sauce.

5. Add the cooked rice noodles, tofu, and sauce to the skillet with the vegetables. Toss everything together until well combined and heated through.

6. Push the noodle mixture to the side of the skillet and pour the beaten eggs into the empty space. Scramble the eggs, then mix them into the noodles.

7. Serve the tofu and vegetable pad thai warm, garnished with chopped peanuts and cilantro.

This dish is a great source of plant-based protein, complex carbs, and a variety of vegetables. The peanut sauce adds a delicious flavor that makes it a satisfying meal for athletes.

85. Chickpea and vegetable tagine with couscous

Ingredients:
- 1 cup uncooked couscous
- 1 tbsp olive oil
- 1 onion, diced
- 3 cloves garlic, minced
- 1 tbsp grated fresh ginger
- 2 tsp ground cumin
- 1 tsp ground coriander
- 1 tsp paprika
- 1/2 tsp ground cinnamon
- 1/4 tsp cayenne pepper (optional)
- 1 (15 oz) can chickpeas, drained and rinsed
- 1 (14 oz) can diced tomatoes
- 2 cups low-sodium vegetable broth
- 2 cups mixed vegetables (such as cauliflower, sweet potato, zucchini)
- Salt and pepper to taste
- Chopped cilantro for garnish

Instructions:

1. Prepare the couscous according to package instructions. Fluff with a fork and set aside.

2. In a large pot or Dutch oven, heat the olive oil over medium heat. Add the onion and sauté for 3-4 minutes until translucent.

3. Add the garlic, ginger, cumin, coriander, paprika, cinnamon, and cayenne (if using). Cook for 1 minute, stirring constantly, until fragrant.

4. Stir in the chickpeas, diced tomatoes, vegetable broth, and mixed vegetables. Bring the mixture to a boil, then reduce heat and simmer for 15-20 minutes, until the vegetables are tender.

5. Season the tagine with salt and pepper to taste.

6. Serve the chickpea and vegetable tagine over the cooked couscous, garnished with chopped cilantro.

This dish is a nutritious and flavorful option for athletes, providing plant-based protein, complex carbs, fiber, and a variety of essential vitamins and minerals. The Moroccan-inspired spices add depth of flavor.

86. Grilled shrimp and vegetable kabobs with quinoa

Ingredients:
- 1 lb large shrimp, peeled and deveined
- 1 zucchini, cut into 1-inch pieces
- 1 red bell pepper, cut into 1-inch pieces
- 1 red onion, cut into 1-inch pieces
- 8 oz mushrooms, halved
- 1 cup uncooked quinoa
- 2 tbsp olive oil
- 2 tbsp lemon juice
- 1 tsp dried oregano
- 1 tsp garlic powder
- Salt and pepper to taste

Instructions:

1. Preheat grill to medium-high heat.

2. In a large bowl, combine the shrimp, zucchini, bell pepper, onion, and mushrooms. Drizzle with olive oil, lemon juice, oregano, garlic powder, salt, and pepper. Toss to coat.

3. Thread the shrimp and vegetables onto skewers, alternating the ingredients.

4. Grill the kabobs for 12-15 minutes, turning occasionally, until the shrimp are opaque and the vegetables are tender.

5. Meanwhile, cook the quinoa according to package instructions. Fluff with a fork.

6. Serve the grilled shrimp and vegetable kabobs over the cooked quinoa.

This dish is packed with lean protein from the shrimp, complex carbs from the quinoa, and a variety of nutrient-dense vegetables. It's a well-balanced and flavorful meal for active individuals.

87. Mediterranean-style baked cod with roasted vegetables

Ingredients:
- 4 (6 oz) cod fillets
- 2 tbsp olive oil, divided
- 1 cup diced zucchini
- 1 cup diced bell peppers
- 1 cup diced red onion
- 2 cloves garlic, minced
- 1 tsp dried oregano
- 1 tsp paprika
- Zest of 1 lemon
- Salt and pepper to taste
- Chopped fresh parsley for garnish

Instructions:

1. Preheat oven to 400°F. Line a baking sheet with parchment paper.

2. In a large bowl, toss the diced zucchini, bell peppers, red onion, and garlic with 1 tbsp of the olive oil. Season with salt and pepper.

3. Spread the seasoned vegetables in a single layer on the prepared baking sheet. Roast for 20-25 minutes, until tender and lightly browned.

4. In a small bowl, combine the remaining 1 tbsp of olive oil, oregano, paprika, lemon zest, salt, and pepper. Rub the mixture over the cod fillets.

5. Place the cod fillets on a separate baking sheet. Bake for 12-15 minutes, until the fish flakes easily with a fork.

6. Serve the baked cod fillets over the roasted Mediterranean vegetables, garnished with chopped fresh parsley.

This dish is a great source of lean protein from the cod, healthy fats from the olive oil, and a variety of nutrient-dense vegetables. It's a well-balanced and flavorful meal for active individuals.

88. Turkey and vegetable stuffed peppers with quinoa

Ingredients:
- 1 cup uncooked quinoa
- 4 bell peppers, halved lengthwise and seeds removed
- 1 lb ground turkey
- 1 cup diced onion
- 1 cup diced bell pepper
- 2 cloves garlic, minced
- 1 tsp dried oregano
- 1 tsp dried basil
- 1/2 tsp red pepper flakes (optional)
- Salt and pepper to taste
- 1 cup shredded mozzarella cheese

Instructions:

1. Cook the quinoa according to package instructions. Fluff with a fork and set aside.

2. Preheat oven to 400°F. Arrange the bell pepper halves in a baking dish.

3. In a large skillet over medium heat, cook the ground turkey, breaking it up as it cooks, until no longer pink, about 5-7 minutes. Drain any excess fat.

4. Add the diced onion, bell pepper, garlic, oregano, basil, red pepper flakes (if using), salt, and pepper to the skillet with the turkey. Cook for 5-7 minutes, until the vegetables are tender.

5. Stir the cooked quinoa into the turkey and vegetable mixture.

6. Spoon the quinoa and turkey filling evenly into the bell pepper halves.

7. Top each stuffed pepper with shredded mozzarella cheese.

8. Bake for 20-25 minutes, until the peppers are tender and the cheese is melted and bubbly.9. Serve the stuffed peppers warm.

This dish is a great source of lean protein, complex carbs, fiber, and essential vitamins and minerals. The bell peppers provide a nutrient-dense vessel for the flavorful quinoa and turkey filling.

89. Tofu and vegetable stir-fry with soba noodles

Ingredients:
- 8 oz soba noodles
- 1 block (14 oz) extra-firm tofu, cubed
- 2 tbsp sesame oil, divided
- 2 cups mixed vegetables (such as broccoli, carrots, snow peas, bell peppers)
- 2 cloves garlic, minced
- 1 tbsp grated fresh ginger
- 2 tbsp low-sodium soy sauce
- 1 tbsp rice vinegar
- 1 tsp honey
- Salt and pepper to taste
- Chopped green onions and toasted sesame seeds for garnish (optional)

Instructions:

1. Cook the soba noodles according to package instructions. Drain and set aside.

2. In a large skillet or wok, heat 1 tbsp of the sesame oil over medium-high heat. Add the cubed tofu and cook for 5-7 minutes, turning occasionally, until lightly browned on all sides. Transfer the tofu to a plate.

3. In the same skillet, heat the remaining 1 tbsp of sesame oil. Add the mixed vegetables, garlic, and ginger. Stir-fry for 5-7 minutes, until the vegetables are tender-crisp.

4. Return the tofu to the skillet. Add the soy sauce, rice vinegar, and honey. Toss to coat everything evenly and heat through.

5. Add the cooked soba noodles to the skillet and toss to combine.

6. Serve the tofu and vegetable stir-fry with soba noodles, garnished with chopped green onions and toasted sesame seeds, if desired.

This dish is a great source of plant-based protein from the tofu, complex carbs from the soba noodles, and a variety of nutrient-dense vegetables. It's a well-balanced and flavorful meal for active individuals.

90. Lentil and vegetable shepherd's pie with mashed cauliflower

Ingredients:
For the Filling:
- 1 cup dry brown or green lentils, rinsed
- 2 cups low-sodium vegetable broth
- 1 tbsp olive oil
- 1 onion, diced
- 2 carrots, diced
- 2 celery stalks, diced
- 3 cloves garlic, minced
- 1 tsp dried thyme
- 1 tsp dried rosemary
- 1 (14 oz) can diced tomatoes
- Salt and pepper to taste

For the Topping:
- 1 head cauliflower, cut into florets
- 2 tbsp unsweetened almond milk
- 1 tbsp olive oil
- Salt and pepper to taste

Instructions:

1. Preheat oven to 375°F.

2. In a medium saucepan, combine the lentils and vegetable broth. Bring to a boil, then reduce heat and simmer for 20-25 minutes, until the lentils are tender. Drain any excess liquid and set aside.

3. In a large skillet, heat the olive oil over medium heat. Add the onion, carrots, celery, and garlic. Sauté for 5-7 minutes, until the vegetables are tender.

4. Stir in the cooked lentils, thyme, rosemary, and diced tomatoes. Season with salt and pepper to taste.

5. Transfer the lentil and vegetable mixture to a 9x13 inch baking dish.

6. In a medium saucepan, cover the cauliflower florets with water and bring to a boil. Reduce heat and simmer for 15-20 minutes, until the cauliflower is very soft. Drain and return to the saucepan.

7. Mash the cauliflower with the almond milk and olive oil. Season with salt and pepper. Spread the mashed cauliflower evenly over the lentil and vegetable filling.

8. Bake for 25-30 minutes, until the topping is lightly browned. Let the shepherd's pie cool for 5-10 minutes before serving.

This dish is a nutritious and satisfying meal for athletes, providing plant-based protein, complex carbs, fiber, and essential vitamins and minerals.

91. Greek-style grilled chicken with quinoa salad

Ingredients:
- 4 boneless, skinless chicken breasts
- 2 tbsp olive oil
- 2 tbsp lemon juice
- 2 tsp dried oregano
- 1 tsp garlic powder
- Salt and pepper to taste

For the Quinoa Salad:
- 1 cup uncooked quinoa, rinsed
- 1 cup cherry tomatoes, halved
- 1 cucumber, diced
- 1/2 red onion, thinly sliced
- 1/4 cup crumbled feta cheese
- 2 tbsp chopped fresh parsley
- 2 tbsp olive oil
- 1 tbsp red wine vinegar
- Salt and pepper to taste

Instructions:

1. In a shallow dish, combine the olive oil, lemon juice, oregano, garlic powder, salt and pepper. Add the chicken breasts and turn to coat both sides. Cover and marinate for 30 minutes to 1 hour.

2. Preheat grill or grill pan to medium-high heat. Grill the chicken for 5-7 minutes per side, until cooked through.

3. While the chicken is grilling, cook the quinoa according to package instructions. Fluff with a fork and let cool slightly.

4. In a large bowl, combine the cooked quinoa, tomatoes, cucumber, red onion, feta and parsley. Drizzle with olive oil and vinegar, then season with salt and pepper. Toss to coat.

5. Serve the grilled chicken over the quinoa salad. Enjoy!

This dish is packed with lean protein, complex carbs, healthy fats and antioxidants - perfect for fueling active athletes. The lemon, oregano and feta give it a delicious Greek-inspired flavor.

92. Baked salmon with mango avocado salsa and brown rice

Ingredients:
For the Salmon:
- 4 (6 oz) salmon fillets
- 2 tbsp olive oil
- 1 tsp garlic powder
- 1 tsp paprika
- Salt and pepper to taste

For the Brown Rice:
- 1 cup uncooked brown rice
- 2 cups low-sodium chicken or vegetable broth

For the Mango Avocado Salsa:
- 1 ripe mango, diced
- 1 avocado, diced
- 1/4 cup diced red onion
- 1 jalapeño, seeded and minced
- 2 tbsp chopped cilantro
- 1 tbsp lime juice
- Salt and pepper to taste

Instructions:

1. Preheat oven to 400°F. Line a baking sheet with parchment paper.

2. Place the salmon fillets on the prepared baking sheet. Drizzle with olive oil and sprinkle with garlic powder, paprika, salt and pepper. Bake for 12-15 minutes, until salmon is cooked through.

3. While the salmon is baking, make the mango avocado salsa. In a medium bowl, gently mix together the mango, avocado, red onion, jalapeño, cilantro and lime juice. Season with salt and pepper.

4. Cook the brown rice according to package instructions, using broth instead of water for extra flavor.

5. Serve the baked salmon over the brown rice, topped with the mango avocado salsa. Enjoy!

This dish is packed with heart-healthy omega-3s from the salmon, complex carbs from the brown rice, and antioxidants and healthy fats from the mango and avocado. It's a nutritious and delicious meal for active athletes.

93. Turkey and vegetable lettuce wraps with peanut sauce

Ingredients:
For the Lettuce Wraps:
- 1 lb ground turkey
- 1 tbsp sesame oil
- 2 cloves garlic, minced
- 1 tbsp grated fresh ginger
- 1 cup shredded carrots
- 1 cup shredded cabbage
- 1/2 cup diced red bell pepper
- 2 tbsp low-sodium soy sauce
- 1 tbsp rice vinegar
- Salt and pepper to taste
- 12-16 large lettuce leaves (such as romaine or bibb)

For the Peanut Sauce:
- 1/4 cup creamy peanut butter
- 2 tbsp low-sodium soy sauce
- 2 tbsp rice vinegar
- 1 tbsp honey
- 1 tsp sesame oil
- 1-2 tbsp water to thin

Instructions:
1. In a large skillet over medium-high heat, cook the ground turkey in sesame oil, breaking it up as it cooks, until no longer pink, about 5-7 minutes.

2. Add the garlic and ginger and cook for 1 minute more until fragrant.

3. Stir in the carrots, cabbage, bell pepper, soy sauce and rice vinegar. Season with salt and pepper. Cook for 2-3 minutes until vegetables are tender.

4. In a small bowl, whisk together all the peanut sauce ingredients, adding water as needed to reach desired consistency.

5. To serve, spoon the turkey and vegetable mixture into the lettuce leaves. Drizzle with the peanut sauce.

This dish is a great source of lean protein from the turkey, fiber and vitamins from the vegetables, and healthy fats from the peanut sauce. The lettuce wraps make it a light but satisfying meal for active athletes.

94. Quinoa and black bean stuffed bell peppers with avocado

Ingredients:
- 4 large bell peppers, halved lengthwise and seeds removed
- 1 cup cooked quinoa
- 1 (15 oz) can black beans, rinsed and drained
- 1 cup diced tomatoes
- 1/2 cup diced onion
- 2 cloves garlic, minced
- 1 tsp cumin
- 1 tsp chili powder
- Salt and pepper to taste
- 1 avocado, diced
- 1/4 cup crumbled feta cheese (optional)
- Chopped cilantro for garnish

Instructions:

1. Preheat oven to 375°F. Place the bell pepper halves cut-side up in a baking dish.

2. In a large bowl, combine the cooked quinoa, black beans, tomatoes, onion, garlic, cumin, chili powder, salt and pepper. Mix well.

3. Spoon the quinoa and black bean mixture evenly into the bell pepper halves.

4. Bake for 25-30 minutes, until the peppers are tender.

5. Remove from oven and top each stuffed pepper with diced avocado and crumbled feta cheese (if using).

6. Garnish with chopped cilantro and serve.

This dish is packed with plant-based protein from the quinoa and black beans, healthy fats from the avocado, and a variety of vitamins and minerals from the bell peppers and other veggies. It's a nutritious and satisfying meal for active athletes.

95. Tofu and vegetable curry with brown rice

Ingredients:
For the Curry:
- 1 block (14 oz) extra-firm tofu, cubed
- 2 tbsp coconut oil
- 1 onion, diced
- 3 cloves garlic, minced
- 1 tbsp grated fresh ginger
- 2 tsp curry powder
- 1 tsp ground cumin

- 1 tsp ground coriander
- 1 tsp turmeric
- 1 cup diced carrots
- 1 cup diced cauliflower florets
- 1 cup diced zucchini
- 1 (13.5 oz) can coconut milk
- 1 cup low-sodium vegetable broth
- 2 tbsp tomato paste
- Salt and pepper to taste
- Chopped cilantro for garnish

For the Brown Rice:
- 1 cup uncooked brown rice
- 2 cups low-sodium vegetable broth

Instructions:

1. Cook the brown rice according to package instructions, using 2 cups of vegetable broth instead of water.

2. In a large skillet or wok, heat the coconut oil over medium-high heat. Add the tofu cubes and cook for 5-7 minutes, turning occasionally, until lightly browned on all sides. Transfer tofu to a plate.

3. In the same skillet, sauté the onion for 3-4 minutes until translucent. Add the garlic and ginger and cook for 1 minute more.

4. Stir in the curry powder, cumin, coriander and turmeric. Cook for 1 minute to toast the spices.

5. Add the carrots, cauliflower and zucchini. Pour in the coconut milk, vegetable broth and tomato paste. Bring to a simmer.

6. Reduce heat to medium-low and let the curry simmer for 10-15 minutes, until vegetables are tender.

7. Gently stir the cooked tofu back into the curry. Season with salt and pepper. Serve the curry over the cooked brown rice, garnished with chopped cilantro.

This curry is packed with plant-based protein from the tofu, complex carbs from the brown rice, and a variety of vitamins and minerals from the vegetables. It's a nutritious and flavorful meal for active athletes.

96. Chickpea and vegetable tikka masala with quinoa

Ingredients:

For the Tikka Masala:
- 1 (15 oz) can chickpeas, rinsed and drained
- 2 tbsp olive oil
- 1 onion, diced
- 3 cloves garlic, minced
- 1 tbsp grated fresh ginger
- 2 tsp garam masala

For the Quinoa:
- 1 cup uncooked quinoa, rinsed
- 2 cups low-sodium vegetable broth

- 1 tsp ground cumin
- 1 tsp paprika
- 1/2 tsp cayenne pepper (optional)
- 1 (14 oz) can diced tomatoes
- 1 cup low-sodium vegetable broth
- 1 cup diced cauliflower florets
- 1 cup diced bell pepper
- 1/2 cup plain Greek yogurt
- Salt and pepper to taste
- Chopped cilantro for garnish

Instructions:

1. Cook the quinoa according to package instructions, using 2 cups of vegetable broth instead of water.

2. In a large skillet or pot, heat the olive oil over medium heat. Add the onion and sauté for 3-4 minutes until translucent.

3. Stir in the garlic, ginger, garam masala, cumin, paprika and cayenne (if using). Cook for 1 minute to toast the spices.

4. Add the chickpeas, diced tomatoes, vegetable broth, cauliflower and bell pepper. Bring to a simmer.

5. Reduce heat to medium-low and let the tikka masala simmer for 10-15 minutes, until vegetables are tender.

6. Remove from heat and stir in the Greek yogurt. Season with salt and pepper.

7. Serve the chickpea and vegetable tikka masala over the cooked quinoa. Garnish with chopped cilantro.

This dish is packed with plant-based protein from the chickpeas, complex carbs from the quinoa, and a variety of vitamins and minerals from the vegetables. The tikka masala sauce provides a flavorful and aromatic element. It's a nutritious and satisfying meal for active athletes.

97. Greek-style baked cod with roasted vegetables and couscous

Ingredients:
- 4 cod fillets (about 6 oz each)
- 2 tbsp olive oil
- 1 lemon, juiced
- 2 tsp dried oregano
- 1 tsp garlic powder
- Salt and pepper to taste
- 2 cups mixed vegetables (such as zucchini, bell peppers, onions, cherry tomatoes), chopped
- 1 cup couscous
- 1 cup vegetable or chicken broth

Instructions:

1. Preheat your oven to 400°F (200°C).

2. In a baking dish, arrange the cod fillets. Drizzle with 1 tbsp of olive oil, lemon juice, oregano, garlic powder, and season with salt and pepper.

3. In a separate baking tray, toss the chopped vegetables with the remaining 1 tbsp of olive oil. Season with salt and pepper.

4. Place both the cod and the vegetables in the oven and bake for 15-20 minutes, or until the cod is flaky and the vegetables are tender.

5. While the cod and vegetables are baking, prepare the couscous. In a saucepan, bring the broth to a boil. Remove from heat, stir in the couscous, cover, and let sit for 5-7 minutes until the couscous is tender and has absorbed all the liquid.

6. Serve the baked cod on a bed of couscous, topped with the roasted vegetables. Enjoy!

This dish is packed with lean protein from the cod, complex carbs from the couscous, and a variety of vitamins and minerals from the roasted vegetables. It's a well-balanced meal that can provide sustained energy for athletes.

98. Turkey and vegetable stir-fry with quinoa

Ingredients:
- 1 lb ground turkey
- 2 tbsp olive oil
- 1 onion, diced
- 3 cloves garlic, minced
- 1 red bell pepper, sliced
- 1 cup broccoli florets
- 1 cup sliced mushrooms
- 1 cup snow peas or snap peas
- 2 tbsp low-sodium soy sauce or tamari
- 1 tbsp rice vinegar
- 1 tsp grated ginger
- 1/2 tsp red pepper flakes (optional)
- Salt and pepper to taste
- 1 cup uncooked quinoa
- 2 cups low-sodium chicken or vegetable broth

Instructions:

1. Cook the quinoa: In a saucepan, bring the broth to a boil. Add the quinoa, cover, and reduce heat to low. Simmer for 15-20 minutes, until quinoa is tender and liquid is absorbed. Fluff with a fork and set aside.

2. In a large skillet or wok, heat the olive oil over medium-high heat. Add the ground turkey and cook, breaking it up with a wooden spoon, until browned and cooked through, about 5-7 minutes.

3. Add the onion and garlic to the skillet and cook for 2-3 minutes, until fragrant.

4. Stir in the bell pepper, broccoli, mushrooms, and snow peas. Cook for 5-7 minutes, until the vegetables are tender-crisp.

5. In a small bowl, whisk together the soy sauce, rice vinegar, ginger, and red pepper flakes (if using). Pour the sauce into the skillet and toss to coat the turkey and vegetables.

6. Serve the turkey and vegetable stir-fry over the cooked quinoa. Season with salt and pepper to taste.

This dish is a great source of lean protein from the turkey, complex carbs from the quinoa, and a variety of vitamins and minerals from the vegetables. It's a well-balanced meal that can provide sustained energy for athletes.

99. Tofu and vegetable pad thai

Ingredients:
- 8 oz rice noodles
- 2 tbsp vegetable oil
- 1 block (14 oz) firm or extra-firm tofu, cubed
- 2 cloves garlic, minced
- 1 cup shredded carrots
- 1 cup bean sprouts
- 1 cup chopped broccoli florets
- 2 eggs, lightly beaten
- 2 tbsp low-sodium soy sauce or tamari
- 2 tbsp rice vinegar
- 1 tbsp honey or maple syrup
- 1 tsp chili-garlic sauce (or to taste)
- 2 tbsp chopped roasted peanuts
- 2 tbsp chopped fresh cilantro
- 1 lime, cut into wedges

Instructions:

1. Soak the rice noodles in hot water for 15-20 minutes, until softened. Drain and set aside.

2. In a large skillet or wok, heat the vegetable oil over medium-high heat. Add the cubed tofu and cook, stirring occasionally, until lightly browned on all sides, about 5-7 minutes. Transfer the tofu to a plate and set aside.

3. In the same skillet, add the garlic and cook for 1 minute, until fragrant. Add the carrots, bean sprouts, and broccoli, and stir-fry for 3-4 minutes, until the vegetables are tender-crisp.

4. Push the vegetables to the side of the skillet and pour the beaten eggs into the empty space. Scramble the eggs, then mix them into the vegetables.

5. Add the cooked noodles, tofu, soy sauce, rice vinegar, honey, and chili-garlic sauce to the skillet. Toss everything together until well combined and heated through.

6. Serve the pad thai hot, garnished with the chopped peanuts, cilantro, and a lime wedge.

This pad thai is a great source of plant-based protein from the tofu, complex carbs from the rice noodles, and a variety of vitamins and minerals from the vegetables. It's a well-balanced meal that can provide sustained energy for athletes.

100. Lentil and vegetable curry with brown rice

Ingredients:
- 1 cup brown rice
- 2 cups low-sodium vegetable broth
- 1 tbsp olive oil
- 1 onion, diced
- 3 cloves garlic, minced
- 1 tbsp grated ginger
- 2 tsp curry powder
- 1 tsp ground cumin
- 1/2 tsp ground coriander
- 1/4 tsp cayenne pepper (or to taste)
- 1 cup red lentils, rinsed
- 1 can (14 oz) diced tomatoes
- 1 cup chopped cauliflower florets
- 1 cup chopped sweet potato
- 1 cup chopped spinach or kale
- 1 cup coconut milk
- Salt and pepper to taste
- Chopped cilantro for garnish

Instructions:

1. Cook the brown rice: In a saucepan, bring the vegetable broth to a boil. Add the brown rice, cover, and reduce heat to low. Simmer for 25-30 minutes, until rice is tender and liquid is absorbed. Fluff with a fork and set aside.

2. In a large skillet or Dutch oven, heat the olive oil over medium heat. Add the onion and cook for 3-4 minutes, until translucent.

3. Stir in the garlic, ginger, curry powder, cumin, coriander, and cayenne. Cook for 1 minute, until fragrant.

4. Add the lentils, diced tomatoes, cauliflower, sweet potato, and coconut milk. Bring to a simmer and cook for 15-20 minutes, until the lentils and vegetables are tender. Stir in the spinach or kale and cook for 2-3 minutes, until the greens are wilted.

5. Season the curry with salt and pepper to taste. Serve the lentil and vegetable curry over the cooked brown rice, garnished with chopped cilantro.

This curry is a great source of plant-based protein from the lentils, complex carbs from the brown rice, and a variety of vitamins and minerals from the vegetables. It's a well-balanced meal that can provide sustained energy for athletes.

Congratulations on completing ***Healthy Cookbook For Athletes: 100 Recipes Balanced Meals for Strength, Stamina, and Speed!***

We hope that this culinary journey has been enriching and enjoyable, providing you with the tools and inspiration to fuel your athletic performance with balanced, nutritious meals. Over the course of these 100 recipes, you've explored a wide array of flavors and ingredients, all designed to support your goals for strength, stamina, and speed.

Your dedication to optimizing your nutrition is commendable, and it's a crucial aspect of achieving peak performance in your athletic endeavors. The knowledge and skills you've gained through these recipes will not only enhance your current training and competitions but also foster lifelong healthy eating habits.

Remember, nutrition is an ongoing journey. Continue to listen to your body, experiment with new foods, and adapt your meals to meet your evolving needs and preferences. Stay curious, keep learning, and enjoy the process of nourishing your body and mind.

We hope this cookbook has inspired you to view food as a powerful tool for enhancing your athletic capabilities and overall well-being. Your commitment to eating balanced, nutrient-rich meals will undoubtedly contribute to your success both on and off the field.

Thank you for choosing ***Healthy Cookbook For Athletes.*** We are honored to have been a part of your journey towards better health and performance. May these recipes continue to fuel your passion, drive your success, and support your pursuit of excellence.

Stay strong, stay energized, and keep pushing your limits!

Warmest regards,

Daisy Robinson